The Origins of Artificial Cranial Formation in Eurasia from the Sixth Millennium B.C. to the Seventh Century A.D.

István Kiszely

Translated from the Hungarian by
Catherine Simán

BAR International Series
(Supplementary) 50
1978

B.A.R.

122, Banbury Road, Oxford, OX2 7BP, England

GENERAL EDITORS

A. R. Hands, B.Sc., M.A., D.Phil.
D. R. Walker, M.A.

B. A. R. International Series (Supplementary) 50, 1978: "The Origins of Artificial Cranial Formation in Eurasia from the Sixth Millenium B. C. to the Seventh Century A.D."

© István Kiszely, 1978

The author's moral rights under the 1988 UK Copyright,
Designs and Patents Act are hereby expressly asserted.

All rights reserved. No part of this work may be copied, reproduced, stored, sold, distributed, scanned, saved in any form of digital format or transmitted in any form digitally, without the written permission of the Publisher.

ISBN 9780860540298 paperback
ISBN 9781407348018 e-book
DOI https://doi.org/10.30861/9780860540298
A catalogue record for this book is available from the British Library
This book is available at www.barpublishing.com

CONTENTS

	Page
List of Illustrations	
List of Tables	
Introduction	1
A short review of the history of the discovery of intentionally formed skulls in Eurasia up to 1878	3
Eridu	7
The custom of intentional head formation in the present-day territory of the U.S.S.R.	13
Intentionally formed skulls in South and South-east Europe	21
Romania	21
Bulgaria	21
Greece	21
Jugoslavia	21
Italy	22
Intentionally formed skulls found in the Carpathian Basin region	23
Intentionally formed skulls from the territory of the Rugii (Lower Austria and Moravia), and the vicinity of Vienna	32
The final areas of expansion of the custom	35
Bohemia	35
Central Germany, Thuringia	36
South Germany, Rhine Valley	37
Tables 1-5	43f.
Bibliography	52
Figures 1-41	77f.

LIST OF ILLUSTRATIONS

Figure		Page
1	Artificially formed skulls from Byblos, Lebanon	77
2	Artificially formed skulls from Eridu (Tell Abu Shahrain), Iraq	78
3	Artificially formed skulls from Eridu (Tell Abu Shahrain), Iraq	79
4	Artificially formed skulls from Eridu (Tell Abu Shahrain), Iraq	80
5	Artificially formed skulls from Eridu (Tell Abu Shahrain), Iraq	81
6	Artificially formed skull in situ, from the Cemetery at Khirokitia, Cyprus	82
7	Sites where artificially formed skulls have been found in the Near East and the Soviet Union	83
8	Artificially formed skulls from Ordzonikidze (Dzaudzhikau), Caucasus	84
9	Artificially formed skulls from the U.S.S.R.	85
10	Sites where artificially formed skulls have been found in Southern and South-Eastern Europe	86
11	Differences between some artificially formed skulls found in Italy (Norma lateralis)	87
12	Artificially formed skulls from Romania, Hungary and Greece	88
13	Sites where artificially formed skulls have been found in the Carpathian Basin	89
14	Artificially formed skulls deriving from South Hungary	90
15	Artificially formed skulls from Southern Hungary	91
16	Artificially formed skulls from Hungary	92
17	Artificially formed skulls from Hungary	93
18	Artificially formed skull viewed along 4 axes, from Fertőszentmiklós, Hungary	94
19	Artificially formed skulls in situ	95

Figure		Page
20	Artificially formed skull from Soponya (Hungary)	96
21	Artificially formed skull from Soponya (Hungary)	97
22	Artificially formed skulls from Hungary	98
23	Artificially formed skulls from Central and Southern Europe	99
24	Artificially formed skulls from Austria	100
25	Sites in the territory of the Rugii and in the Vienna region where artificially formed skulls have been found	101
26	Artificially formed skulls from Austria	102
27	Artificially formed skulls from Moravia	103
28	Artificially formed skulls from Moravia.	104
29	Artificially formed skulls from Novy Saldorf, Moravia	105
30	Artificially formed skulls from Velatice, Moravia	106
31	Artificially formed skulls from Czechoslovakia	107
32	Sites in Central and Western Europe where artificially formed skulls have been found	108
33	Artificially formed skulls from Germany	109
34	Artificially formed skulls from Germany	110
35	Methods of artificially forming the skulls of the newborn children used in Eurasia	111
36	Skull changes arising from artificial cranial formation (after H. Hellmuth)	112
37	Measurements taken to determine the extent of cranial formation	113
38	Artificially formed skull from Hács-Béndekpuszta (Hungary)	114
39	The reconstruction of the face of the artificially formed skull from Hács-Béndekpuszta (Hungary)	115
40	X-ray photograph of the artificially formed skull from Tamási-Adorjánpuszta, Hungary	116
41	A Mangbetu woman with artificially formed head (H. Bernatzik)	117

LIST OF TABLES

Table		Page
1.	Artificially deformed skulls from Eridu (Tell Abu Shahrain)	43
2.	Measurements of artificially deformed skulls from Szentes-Bökény, Hungary	45
3.	Measurements of artificially deformed skulls from the Roman cemetery at Intercisa (Dunaujváros), Hungary	46
4.	Measurements of artificially deformed skulls from the cemeteries at Burgstall (Austria), Rácalmás and Fertőszentmiklós (Hungary)	48
5.	Measurements of artificially deformed skulls from Nikitsch and Steinbrunn	50

INTRODUCTION

The custom of head "deformation" has been practiced in all parts of the world (Europe, Asia, Africa, Oceania and America) and at different historical periods independently or through migration or cultural exchange, by means of bandages, pillows or fastening the head to the cradle with a cap. The method of formation was different in different cases. The new form of the head corresponded to the contemporary ideal of beauty, and the direction of the formation coincided with that of the original form. Thus the custom of head formation in Eurasia came into existence among the long-headed people, so the newly formed head was long, while in Peru the originally short head was made even shorter, the long one even longer. Usually the natural characteristics were emphasized since they were considered beautiful. The aim was therefore to make the head more beautiful and nobler, and so the word "deformation" is misleading and the expression "formation" should be used instead.

The first "abnormal" skull to be found in Europe came from Grafenegg (Austria) in 1820, the next one was from Atzgersdorf (Austria) in 1846. The scientific description of the Atzgersdorf skull was published by J. Fitzinger in 1853. In 1877 and in 1878 J. Lenhossék, an anatomist from Budapest, summed up the finds unearthed so far in an essay. The first finds were ascribed to the Cimmerians by P. Broca, to the Avars by J. Fitzinger, to the Alans by M. Smirnov, and so on. The similar finds from other parts of the world were summed up by A. Grosse in Paris under the title "Essais sur les déformations artificielles du crâne". K. Baer wrote a monograph about the finds discovered in the Crimea: "Die Makrokephalen im Boden der Krym und Österreichs" (1860).

The number of finds was increasing rapidly, while their proper ethnic place became more and more uncertain. Carl Ernst von Baer, after the discovery of the Csongrád and Székelyudvarhely (Hungary) "deformed" skulls wrote the following to J. Lenhossék: "if any further macrocephalic skull should be discovered in Hungary, it should be mentioned in the history of the country". In the first decades of this century L. Bartucz wrote that "the custom of intentional head formation can be related to the whole of the ethnic anthropology of Eurasia".

Most of the skeletons with intentionally formed skulls belonged to the Ostrogoths, the Alans, the Sarmations and the Quadi of the Migration Period. The sudden invasion of these peoples into Central and Southern Europe may have been strongly connected with that of the Huns, which gave rise to the theory that the intentional head formation had been introduced by the Huns. The existence of this theory up till now is due to the lack of a summary of recent finds. Many of these finds in Europe and South-West Asia are older than the Huns. On the other hand no intentionally formed skull has been found in the "best" Hun cemeteries. These facts have led to the weakening of this theory, until it has lost its validity.

All the intentionally formed skulls that have been found cannot be described in this paper as their number is increasing rapidly from year to year, now reaching a thousand. The aims of this paper are as follows:

1. description of the especially important finds;
2. ascribing the finds to peoples;
3. the definition of the possible origin and mode of diffusion of the South-West Asian and European custom of intentional head formation in the light of new discoveries.

A SHORT REVIEW OF THE HISTORY OF THE DISCOVERY OF INTENTIONALLY FORMED SKULLS IN EURASIA UP TO 1878

Many of the ancient authors mention the "makrokephaloi" living in Asia. Anthropologists in the last century did not ascribe the custom of head formation to the Huns, being aware of the ancient references to head-forming peoples of South-West Asia and the Caucasus written long before the time of the Huns.

Herodotos in about 450 B.C., calls the head-forming peoples "makrones". The custom is also mentioned by Heracleitos (534-475 B.C.), and by Hippocrates (460-377 B.C.), calling them "makrokephaloi". Hippocrates mentions them in Liber Aeribus Aquis et Locis,[14]

καὶ πρῶτον περὶ τῶν Μακροκεφάλων.τούτων γὰρ οὐκ ἔστιν ἄλλο ἔθνος ὁμοίας τὰς κεφαλὰς ἔχον οὐδέν·τὴν μὲν γὰρ ἀρχὴν ὁ νόμος αἰτιώτατος ἐγένετο τοῦ μήκεος τῆς κεφαλῆς,νῦν δὲ καὶ ἡ φύσις συμβάλλεται τῷ νόμῳ.τοὺς γὰρ μακροτάτην ἔχοντας τὴν κεφαλὴν γενναιοτάτους ἡγέονται.ἔχει δὲ περὶ νόμου ὧδε·τὸ παιδίον ὁκόταν γένηται τάχιστα,τὴν κεφαλὴν αὐτου ἔτι ἀπαλὴν ἐοῦσαν μαλθακοῦ ἐόντος ἀναπλάσσουσι τῇσι χερσὶ καὶ ἀναγκάζουσιν ἐς τὸ μῆκος αὔξεσθαι δεσμά τε προσφέροντες καὶ τεχνήματα ἐπιτήδεια,ὑφ'ὧν τὸ μὲν σφαιροειδὲς τῆς κεφαλῆς κακοῦται,τὸ δὲ μῆκος αὔξεται.

Apollonius Rhodios (c. 295-215 B.C.) calls them "makrones", "makrokephaloi", their heads being mostly abnormally long. Strabo (63-c. 7 B.C.) calls them "makrokephaloi" and characterises the Caucasian peoples as follows:

τινὰς δ'ἐπιτηδεύειν φασίν,ὅπως ὡς μακροκεφαλώτατοι φανοῦνται,καὶ προπεπτωκότες τοῖς μετώποις,ὥσθ'ὑπερκύπτειν τῶν γενείων.

Later several other authors mention these Asian people, for example Pliny the Younger in c. 25 A.D., who calls them "makrones".

The first macrocephalic skull from Austria was discovered at Feuersbrunn, near Grafenegg, in 1820, in a row of graves. It was described by A. Retzius, In 1846 another skull was unearthed near Vienna at Atzgersdorf (near Liesing) from under a tumulus. This macrocephalic skull was described by J. Fitzinger. A further find from Austria came from a limestone cave on Calvary

Hill at Baden, near Vienna, between 1823 and 1829. This find was described by G. Rasoumovsky, but J. Fitzinger could not find it some years later, so its scientific publication was impossible. G. Rasoumovsky wrote about the skull:

> "Le front est plus court, le dessus où le sommet est plus ecrasé. Le crâne entière est plus renversé en arrière...La ligne faciale est très inclinée...La tête parait plus courte... les sutures du crâne sont souvent découppées très elegamment...Les os du sommet sont si minées...."

Elsewhere in Central and Western Europe the first skeleton with an intentionally formed skull was found in 1853 at Harnham Hill, in a grave near Salisbury by J. Akerman, J. Davis and F. Barnard. In the same year another skeleton with an intentionally formed skull was found in Villy (Savoy, near Regnier) in a grave of the Old Frankish period, that is to say of Charlemagne's time. It was described by H. Grosse in 1853. A macrocephalic skull was also discovered in Switzerland at Chesaux near Lausanne in Bel-Aire in the 1850s. F. Trojon writes about it:

> "More than 300 graves, lying in three layers one above the other, had been opened, the lowest of which, containing this macrocephalic skull, proved to date from the 5th century".

A macrocephalic skull has been unearthed in an Old Frankish cemetery in Niederholm (Germany) between Mainz and Alzey on the River Rhine in 1862, described by A. Ecker. One found in the Ursula Church in Köln in 1866 was published by A. Schaffhausen. According to him, it "belonged to a Hun, a persecutor of Saint Ursula who was later martyred".

The first intentionally formed skull to come from Hungary, the 11th from Europe, was unearthed at Csongrád in 1867. The second one was found at Székelyudvarhely in 1875. The former was described by J. Lenhossék and the latter by M. Steinburg and later by J. Lenhossek. According to the latter, both skulls date from the 5th century and should be grouped with the Atzgersdorf skull. He described the method of formation of the Csongrád skull as follows (op.cit. p. 64):

> "A hard plate was pushed on the occipital bone, and ribbons were drawn from the forehead to the plate on both sides through the back Casser fontanels, pulled tight and fastened".

The earliest finds of the Eastern head-forming peoples were discovered at the end of the 18th century in the Crimea and the Caucasus. C. Seidlitz in the Caucasus and G. Radde and Sh. Siepura at Tbilisi unearthed 10 intentionally formed skulls, while F. Bayer found skeletons with similar skulls at Samtkharov in Crimea, an area mentioned by Hippocrates (XXXIV... "qui vero ad dextram hyberni ortus solis usque ad Maetidem paludem habitant").

The first "macrocephalic" skull from the Crimea was given to J. Blumenbach by G. Asch, who referred to its possible "Tartaric" origin. J. Blumenbach described it in 1790 under the title "Cranium asiatae makrocephali". The next finds were published by Dubois de Montpereux in 1832 and Rathke in 1833, followed by J. Blumenbach (1833), A. Aschik (in Baer's essay) and K.

Baer (1860). The skulls were sent from the Kertch Peninsula to St. Petersburg, then to Berlin (K. Meyer, 1850), to Bonn (H. Schaffhausen, 1976) and to Paris (G. Grosse).

Regarding the Crimean finds J. Lenhossek ascribed the custom of intentional head formation as follows (p. 82):

> "...Such a great number of intentionally formed macrocephalic skulls found in the Crimea might show, according to K. Baer, that a group of people must have existed, which, as Hippocrates mentions, considered it ennobling to deform the head of the new-born children with bandages and by other means. Now if we consider that the skeletons were found in large numbers and in groups in the Crimea while in Europe there are only a few scattered examples, we can conclude that it is very probable that they must have belonged to a people living in the Crimea".

J. Fitzinger excludes the possibility of ascribing the custom to the Huns, and doubts if Attila's head had ever been intentionally formed:

> "...There is little force in Jordanes description of Attila, the former having, according to Priscus, spent a long time in Attila's camp with the Greek legislators. Jordanes, who knew Attila personally, wrote of him: 'forma brevis, lato pectore, capite grandiori, minutis oculis, rarus barba, canis aspersus, simo naso teter colore originis suae signa restituens'. From this description it is clear that Attila had a large head, but it does not lead to the conclusion that it must have been macrocephalic".

P. Broca ascribed the custom of intentional head formation to the "Cimmerians" living in the neighbourhood of the Scythians in the Crimea in 114 B.C. P. Broca wrote a letter to J. Lenhossék on April 27th, 1877, mentioning Herodotos's "makronoi" in it:

> "...Herodotos mentions the makronoi twice saying that they constituted a part of the Persian Empire, and in Book II, 104, he says that they and the Syrians learnt the custom of circumcision from their neighbours living in Colchis on the banks of the Thermodon and Parthenios...Herodotus' Cimmerians retreated to Asia Minor through the Caucasus...."

J. Lenhossék had B. Lengyel, a university chemist, examine the proportions of the organic and inorganic constituents in the Csongrád and Székelyudvarhely macrocephalic skulls, and then compared the data with that of other, well dated, skulls. With the help of the examinations, carried out by combustion, the theory of which was similar to that of the present absolute dating method of derivatography, he stated that the skulls, discovered in graves with no grave goods, came from the 6th century A.D. "from peoples about which historians know next to nothing" (p. 122).

J. Lenhossek with these studies settled the matter and it took another hundred years for the question to be reopened. The thesis of his monographic summary, based on relatively few and archaeologically ill-determined finds, was as follows:

1. People with intentionally formed heads cannot be identified with the Huns.
2. They arrived in Central and Western Europe from the Crimea a little earlier than the 6th century B.C.
3. The custom arrived in the Crimea from South-Western Asia (Near East) partly through the Caucasus and partly through Asia Minor.
4. The proper ethnic relations of this custom are still unknown.

After a hundred years, in the light of new finds, we can verify J. Lenhossék's statements and can locate the origins of the custom in Asia.

More and more intentionally "deformed" skulls are discovered today in South-West Asia. They are dated to the 6th century B.C. by archaeological, stratigraphical and radiocarbon dating methods. Possibly the practice of head formation came into existence or arrived in South-West Asia at this time. If G. Bräuer's oral information that an intentionally formed skull of the 8th-6th millennia has been found in Mumba cave (Ethiopia) is supported by dating methods and it is scientifically published, it can be presumed that this strange custom arrived in South-West Asia from Africa. This would explain the custom of later head formation in Africa, its appearance in Egypt, and would give us the origins of the appearance of intentionally formed skulls in South-West Asia. If this dating examination does not take place, and if no more recent finds are revealed from earlier times than those in South-West Asia, we must presume that the custom had its origin somewhere in the Near East. In this case the date of the appearance of this custom is uncertain, but it must be placed before the Neolithic, as it is already detectable in the early Neolithic cemetery at Khirokitia (Cyprus).

The first finds from South-West Asia were discovered on the eastern Mediterranian coast of Asia, and the custom penetrated into Mesopotamia and Persia. In the latter territory it survived until the invasion of the Huns; the first "Hun" intentionally formed skulls belong to the Iranian racial type. At the same time the custom became widespread in Asia Minor and in the Caucasus, being practised in the latter territory up to the present dat. An early infiltration (about 2,300 B.C.) into South-East Europe is detectable from the Black Sea or straight from the Caucasus. It became customary in the Crimea before our era among people who, invaded by the Huns, fled to Central Europe in the first centuries of our era.

<u>South-West Asia is therefore to be considered the first centre of intentional head formation</u> in Eurasia in prehistoric and in historic times.

<u>Tell es-Sultan (Jericho)</u> (Jordan). Fragments of skeletons have been unearthed dating from the 8th-4th millennia. The bones were badly preserved in the soil, but some longitudinally formed skulls were found in the upper pre-ceramic layer. According to Kurth's paper (1973) and oral information there were approximately 10 skeletons with formed heads, their date being as yet uncertain. Possibly they date from the 7th-6th millennia B.C.

From <u>Khirokitia</u>, in southern Cyprus, several intentionally formed skulls dating back to the 6th millennium have been reported (Khirokitia period 1, 5,800-4,950 B.C.). Some of them are flattened on the occipital bone, the others have been lengthened by encircling bandages. The finds were published by J. Angel (1953) and G. Kurth (1958). After the restoration of the badly preserved skulls they seem to have belonged to 11 persons (or 43, according to G. Kurth). A re-examination of these skulls has been made by the author.

From Enkombi, Melia and Bambuola 27 skulls with occipital and circular "deformation" have been reported. They date from prehistoric times to the Iron Age.

The intentionally formed skull from Byblos (Lebanon) dated from the first half of the 4th millennium B.C. (H. Contenson, 1965). In the 205 graves in the cemetery, 42 anthropologically measurable skulls were recovered, 21 of which were intentionally formed. Seven skulls were published by H. Vallois in 1937. Most of them belonged to women and girls, some of them to men. The anthropological examination was carried out by M. Ozbek (1974). The method of formation was frontal-occipital, using, presumably, two bandages in two directions. As only a few burials had intentionally formed heads, it is possible that two groups of peoples lived and were buried here (H. Vallois and D. Ferembach, 1962, and M. Sauter, 1945).

At Seyh Höyük (Tell es-Sheik) in Syria on a site with deposits from the Eneolithic to the Iron Age, badly preserved intentionally formed skulls have been found. They were published by M. Senyürek and S. Tunakal in 1951. M. Cappieri ascribed them to the Mediterranian type, resembling the population of Jemdet Nasr, Tépé Gawra, Assur, Al-Ubaid and Ur. The number of the Syrian finds (Seyh Höyük or Tell es-Sheik) is three, all of them women. Their age is approximately the same as that of the Byblos find (Eneolithic).

At Erenkiöi, South-West of Bigha (Dardanelles), Turkey, an extremely "deformed" skull has been found. Neither the circumstances of its finding nor its date are known. It was described by A. Weisbach in 1882 and mentioned by E. Dingwall in 1931.

ERIDU (Tell Abu Shahrain)

Eridu (present-day Tell Abu Shahrain) is in the South-West of Iraq, west of Basra, south-west of An Nasiriya, in the Shamiya desert. It used to be a wealthy trading city on the coast of the Persian Gulf but now it is an insignificant settlement 20 kilometres from the sea.

The Babylonian Genesis says of Eridu:

> "All the Lands were Sea,
> then Eridu was made".

The history of Eridu goes back to the Al'Ubaid period. Its inhabitants lived by fishing; their harbour was the "New Moon" in the south-western part of the city, being rather a tidal lake drained by the recession of the Persian Gulf leaving a fertile marsh, whose water might, perhaps, have been replenished by an outlying channel of the Euphrates. In the Uruk period there was still plentiful evidence of Eridu's importance. From the beginning of the historical period, Eridu no longer appears to have been a populous settlement. Due to the continued recession of the Gulf and the consequent desiccation of the surrounding country or to some other cause, such as a change in the course of the Euphrates, a great part of the site seems to have been abandoned for long periods and its ruined buildings were buried beneath drifting sand. From the third dynasty of Ur, Eridu was not a city but a complex of religious buildings raised high above the surrounding plain on an artificial platform. The Sumerians and the Babylonians worshipped Ea here, the god of wisdom and patron of craftsmen and artisans. He was the father of Marduk and the principal deity of the Sea-People, and it was also he, after whom a city, Dur-Ea, and a king, Ea-gamil, took their names.

The first written source which mentions Eridu is from the time of Ur-Nanshi, who was the founder of the Lagash Dynasty (2,500 B.C.). In the time of the Third Ur Dynasty, Eridu had already been desiccated and was uninhabited. Ur-Nammu, the founder of the Third Dynasty, cut a new channel to the Euphrates to bring water in order that the area could be repeopled. It was also he who built Enki's Temple. Nabuchadnezzar I called himself the "Governor of Eridu" at the end of the 2nd millennium. At the beginning of the 1st millennium Eridu was already an inhabited city or a holy place. The Assyrian king Sargon regarded Eridu's occupation as a triumph in 710 B.C.

Archaeological excavations at Eridu were started in December 1946 under Sayid Mohammed Ali Mustafa's leadership. The first season lasted from 24th December 1946 to 24th March 1947. First the site was located and then the eastern part of the ziggurat was excavated and a building of the Third Dynasty was uncovered, containing rich ornamentation, votive pottery, and a distinctive type of spouted jar containing the bones of animals (Fuad Safar). Not a single burial was found during the first season of the excavations.

The second season ran from the last week of November 1947 to March 1948 under the leadership of Sayid Fuad Safar, who wrote that beside the ziggurat

> "our attention was next directed to the area outside the retaining-wall which supported the Third Dynasty acropolis; and here on the north-western side of the mound, we made a most important discovery. This was a cemetery of the late Al'Ubaid period, contemporary in all probability with Temples VI and VII found in the previous season. In this part of the site there was a deposit of Al'Ubaid occupational debris, about one metre deep, but with a conspicuous absence of building as though we were dealing with the outskirts of the actual settlement. Under this debris, which demonstrably antedated them, the graves were sunk into the clean, wind-drifted sand beneath. They contained liben "boxes", filled with earth after the interment, and sealed with a platform of the same bricks which sometimes considerably overlapped the length and breadth of the actual grave. Like the principal buildings in the main mound they were oriented towards the north west....
> An interesting and unusual practice was that of burying more than one member of the family in the same grave. The bones of the earlier burials were often disturbed in the process, and sometimes quite carelessly pushed aside...It should be dated to the culmination phase of the Al'Ubaid period (this period dates from 4,500-3,800 B.C.). During the course of the season more than two hundred graves were excavated, while soundings made in order to determine the limits of

> the cemetery suggested that it must altogether contain at least a thousand graves...It is not probable, however, that it was in use for any length of time, since all the graves appeared to have been sunk from approximately the same occupational level...
>
> The only slightly unusual feature in the cemetery was the tendency to use rich reddish-brown paint instead of the conventional black" (Fuad Safar, 1948).

A great number of graves were uncovered but the bones were few and damaged. Only a few more or less well preserved skulls survived which were saturated with wax on the spot. Although Charlotte Otten, an anthropologist from the University of Chicago, emphasised the importance of the skeletons during her three days' visit on the site, neither further excavations nor detailed anthropological examination have taken place. Miss Otten wrote (1948):

> "with one possible exception, all of the nine skulls appear to have suffered distortion due to the earth above the burials".

And later:

> "there is apparently no intentional skull deformation, but this point will become more certain after restoration of the skulls...Even upon such cursory examination, it is possible to make a superficial comparison with Sir Arthur Keith's several later Early Dynastic skulls from Al'Ubaid".

When Fuad Safar called her attention to the fact that more than a thousand graves were still unexcavated, Miss Otten wrote:

> "this means, that material is available for a definitive study of a past population such has seldom if ever been equalled. This study could not only identify the range of physical characteristics of the carriers of Ubaid culture, but could provide a clean point of reference upon which further studies of related groups might hinge. It would certainly supplement, and might confirm or disprove theories relating to the early migrations of peoples in the Cradle of Civilisation"... "A through study of this extremely important material could not be other than a milestone in the progress of racial and anthropometric knowledge" (p. 127).

In Sumer, C. Coon (University of Pennsylvania) published his views on the finds. He did not notice the importance of the finds or their being intentionally formed:

> "All the crania had been deformed in one fashion or another, presumably after burial, by earth pressure...This has made them look superficially like certain Maya Indian crania, deformed intentionally in infancy".

Later G. Kurth examined the skulls (1973) realising the intentional formation of them.

> "Die meisten Schädel sind mehr oder weniger erddeformiert, dazu kommt teilweise künstliche Deformation durch Binden, die ebenso,

> wie in Byblos und Jericho die Schädel eher verlängert haben dürften.
> Die vielfach ungewöhnlich schräge Stirn spricht für intravitale Einflüsse" (p. 95.)

In 1977, working on the bone material discovered in Iraq, Donnie Georg and I restored and examined, as far as circumstances made it possible, the bones of the skeletons found at Eridu and preserved in the Iraq Museum in Baghdad. The excavations at Eridu will probably be continued with the collaboration of experts, with the aim of identifying the largest known ancient population of Mesopotamia.

1st skull (labelled No. 1).

A 55 year-old woman's skull with the left temporal area missing. The forehead is low, the nose somewhat projecting, the maxillary part projecting to the sides. It is close to the Iranian Highland type. The skull has been medium "deformed" with encircling bandages. Its anthropological characteristics: dolichocranial, chamae-orthocranial, metriocranial, medium wide forehead, eurymetopic, orthognathous, mesoprosopic, mesene, chamaecranic, mesorrhine, brachystaphyline, mesuranic, fundamental frontal process symmetrically medium wide nasal cavity, rounded rectangular orbits, medium deep fossa canina, tubercled genial process, high, V-form palate, straight sutura palatina, os incae bipartitum, several sutural bones on both sides. Occlusion: labidont. Abrasion of the teeth: 4. Past signs of radiculitis on the upper tooth on the right side. Mesodontes.

2nd skull (labelled No. 2).

The whole skull of a 25 year old man. The skull suffered secondary pressure in the earth, but it left the form of the cranium unchanged. The skull is of negroid character and bears the traces of rather considerable formation. Anthropological characteristics: dolichocranial, chamaecranial, tapeinocranial, narrow forehead, eurymetopic, alveolar prognathia, euryprosopic, euryen, chamaeconchic, chamaerrhine, leptostaphyline, dolichuranic. The lowness of the orbits is due to the secondary pressure. The form of the skull is sphaenoides. Phaenoprosopia, phaenozygia, medium large tubera parietalia, curvo-occipital, thick orbital margins, rounded rectangular orbits, small and straight nasal bone, the nasal cavity is wide below, fossa praenasalis, the zygomatic processes stand out slightly on the sides, the genial process is low pyramid, U-formed palate, many ossa suturarum. Occlusion: stegodont. Megadontes. The upper 3rd molars are erupting.

3rd skull (labelled 116).

Nearly the whole skull of a 35 year-old man, the left maxillary part is a bit fractured. It belongs to the Irano-Afghan type with some robust-Mediterranian influence. The skull is slightly plagiocranic due to secondary pressure in the earth. It was slightly formed in lifetime, this being clearest on the forehead. Anthropological characteristics: doliocranial, chamaecranial, tapeinocranial, narrow forehead, metriometopic, orthognathous, alveolar prognathia, leptoprosopic, leptorene, mesoconchic, leptorrhine, leptostaphyline, dolichuranic. The form of the skull: birdsoides. Phaenoprosopia, phaenozygia, small tubera parientalia, wide sutura sphaenoparietales, thick orbital margins, medium high orbits, medium large nasal bone, symmetrically narrow apertura piriformis, slight fossa praenasalis, zygomatic processes slightly stand out, U-formed and high palate, os incae monopartitum, many ossa suturarum. Occlusion: labidont. Signs of radiculitis on the lower 7th tooth on the right side. Scale on the teeth.

4th skull (labelled 181).

The complete skull of a 40 year old man. The right maxillary part is somewhat fractured, and a part of the base is missing. It belongs to the South-Iraqian type, which inhabits the territory even today. The skull was formed with circular bandages in lifetime. A slight deformation is due to the earth pressure. Anthropological characteristics: hyperdolichocranial, chamaecranial, tapeino-metriocranial, narrow forehead, eurymetopic, orthognathous, euryprosopic, euryen-mesorene, meso-hypsichonchic, mesorrhine, brachyuranic. The form of the skull: birdsoides. Phaenoprosopia, phaenozygia, very small tubera parietalia, rounded rectangular orbits of slanting oval form, apertura piriformis is wide below, the lower part is anthropine. Medium filled fossa canina, the zygomatic processes stand out slightly on the sides, the genial process is low pyramid, the palate is very high. Occlusion: labidont. Mesodontes.

5th skull (labelled III).

The fragmentary skull of a 55 year-old man. The right frontal and some of the parietal parts and also the left mandibula are missing. The skull suffered slight pressure in the earth. Typologically it belongs to the Iranian Highland type characterised with strong alveolar prognathia. The head was considerably formed with circular bandages. Anthropological characteristics: dolicho-mesocranial, chamaecranial, tapeinocranial, medium wide forehead, eurymetopic, orthognathous, slight alveolar prognathia, mesoprosopic, mesorene, mesoconchic, chamaerrhine, mesostaphyline, brachyuranic. The form of the skull: sphaenoides-birdsoides. Phaenoprosopia, phaenozygia, small tubera parietalia, no protuberantia occipitalis externa, thick orbital margins, slanting orbits, apertura piriformis wide below, the lower part is anthropin, medium deep fossa canina, zygomatic processes slightly standing out on the sides, U-formed palate, straight sutura palatina. Occlusion: labidont. Radiculitis on the lower 7th tooth on the right side. The upper 3rd tooth (canine) has been removed in lifetime.

6th skull (labelled N or X_1).

Probably the skull of a 60 year old man, with a broken lower jaw. The pressure of the earth has deformed the line of the orbits, and the face has become low. Disregarding this deformation the skull can be grouped in the Irano-Afghan race type. The skull has in lifetime been formed. The measurements taken of the skull are of dubious value because of the secondary deformation. Anthropological characteristics: dolico-mesocranial, chamaecranial, tapeinocranial, medium wide forehead, eurymetopic, orthognathous, euryen, hypsiconchic, mesostaphyline, brachyuranic. The form of the skull: sphaenoides. Wide sutura sphaenoparietalis, curvooccipital, thick orbital margins, high orbits, symmetrically medium wide apertura piriformis, slight sulcus praenasalis, narrow zygomatics, the zygomatic processes are slightly standing out on the sides, the genial process is tubercled and pyramidal, sutura palatina curving backwards, os epiptericum on sutura sagittalis, spare bones on sutura lambdoidea on both sides. Mesodontes. The upper three molars in the left side have fallen out in lifetime, the ridge is closed.

7th skull (labelled IV).

Calotte and lower jaw of a 25 year old man. The skull belongs to the "classical Mediterranian" type. The intentional head formation is considerable, and perhaps was made with a pillow fastened on the forehead. Anthropological characteristics: mesocranial, chamaecranial, tapeinocranial, medium wide forehead, eurymetopic. The cranial bones are medium thick, the form of the skull is sphaenoides. Small tubera parietalia, narrow sutura sphaenoparietalis, curvo-occipital, very thin orbital margins. The genial process is medium high pyramid. The foramen occipitale magnum is assymmetrical. Many ossa along sutura sagittalis and sutura lambdoidea. Occlusion: labidont. Caries superficialis on three teeth. Mesodontes.

8th skull (no label or labelled X_2).

The highly fractured but nearly total calotte of a 55 year old man. It belongs to a rather robust type. The intentional head formation is very considerable, the nose has flattened in the course of it. The forehead has been formed with double bandage. Anthropological characteristics: dolichocranial orthocranial, metriocranial, medium narrow forehead, eurymetopic, mesoconchic, the gnathions stand out far on both sides, the genial process is feminine. The cranial bones are thick, the form of the skull is sphaenoides-rhomboides. Small tubera parietalia, narrow sutura sphaenoparietalia. The occipital bone is flat due to the formation. There is a torus-like tubercle on tubera nuchae. Medium thick orbital margins, the orbits are rounded rectangular, the nasal bone is straight, the end of it slightly curved, the nasal cavity is symmetrically wide or medium wide, fossa canina medium deep, the zygomatic processes slightly stand out on the sides. There are many ossa on the sutura lambdoidea. Occlusion: labidont. The abbrasion of the teeth is great, the middle teeth are worn till the stump. The second lower incisive on the right side has fallen out in lifetime.

Two further skulls found at Eridu showed no signs of intentional formation. The one labelled II belonged to a 25 year old woman of the "gracil-Mediterranian" type, the other labelled X_3 is the lower jaw of a 50 year old man, who is likely to have belonged to the Irano-Afghan type.

We do not know who inhabited Eridu as yet. Their proper ethnic grouping is still a subject for debate. According to Seaton Lloyd

> "Abu Shahrain is too small to represent the capital of a city-state, and indeed no dynasty of kings is known to have ruled there...we suggest that an original prehistoric shrine had been perpetuated by its repeated reconstruction".

According to Cramer (1944)

> "at the time of the Sumerian invasion much of the land between the Tigris and the Euphrates River was no doubt inhabited by the Semites ...."

E. Speiser writes:

> "the Sumerians cannot be the first inhabitants of Mesopotamia because the oldest cities have non-Sumerian names..."

Seaton Lloyd remarks again that

> "we should now perhaps give fuller consideration to the significance of our new archaeological discoveries at Eridu, in relation to the perennial investigation of Sumerian origin..."

According to Frankfort (1932)

> "the earliest material culture of Southern Mesopotamia must already by called Sumerian".

The bones, though few in number, prove the following:

1. Eridu's population was heterogeneous in about 4,000-3,500 B.C.

2. A population, later called "typical Sumerian", was already present at Eridu.

3. A population with negroid characteristics was already living in the southern part of Mesopotamia in about 4,000 B.C.

4. Intentional head formation of new-born children was a general custom among the early inhabitants of Eridu, disregarding sex and race; it hints at earlier origins.

5. Though no intentional head formation is detectable later among the negroid people in the Near East, it is possible that the origin of the custom is connected with the appearance of negroid people in this area.

6. Further excavations at Eridu may shed light on the origin of the custom of head formation and also that of the first inhabitants of Mesopotamia.

THE CUSTOM OF INTENTIONAL HEAD FORMATION IN THE PRESENT-DAY TERRITORY OF THE USSR

Most of the intentionally formed skulls have been discovered east of the Carpathian Basin in the area between the Pamir-Alai, the Tienshan and western Siberia. No such finds have been found east of this area or north or west of a line drawn between the upper part of the Isim River and the upper part of the Don River. Three "centres" can be distinguished: the Caucasian one, another north of the Black Sea and the Caspian Sea, and lastly the Crimea and areas north of it. The age of the intentionally formed skulls moves on a larger and larger time-scale so the proper ethnical grouping becomes more and more hypothetical.

The catalogue of published sites follows J. Werner's list (1956); some more recent data from later publications are added. Unfortunately, J. Werner's transcriptions and references are not correct and his maps are superficial and of little use. Many of the sites mentioned are marked on the map, fig. 7.

1. <u>Skeletons with intentionally formed skulls from the territory of Pamir-Alai, Tienshan, western Siberia and Central Asia</u>

    1. <u>Kirchin</u> (on the northern shore of the Isik-köl). Skeletons of 65 women and 68 men. Published by A. Bernstam, 1952.

    2. <u>Kizart</u> (Kochkovsky Valley, Djumgal, Tienshan). 6 graves. Published by A. Bernstam, 1952.

    3. <u>Alamishik</u> (on Marim River, Central Tienshan). 12 graves. Published by A. Bernstam, 1952.

    4. <u>Burmachap</u> (Arpa Valley, Central Tienshan). Numerous graves. Published by A. Bernstam, 1952.

    5. <u>Maasha</u> (Alai Valley, North-West of Kara-köl, Pamir). Numerous graves, all containing intentionally formed skulls. Published by A. Bernstam, 1952.

    6. <u>Kisil-Tuu</u> (Alai Valley, North-West of Kara-köl, Pamir). Numerous graves, all containing intentionally formed skulls. Published by A. Bernstam, 1952.

    7. <u>Kenkol</u> (in the Talas Valley). 23 intentionally formed skulls were excavated during the excavations in 1938 and 1939. 13 of them belonged to men, 8 to women and 2 to children. Published by V. Ginzburg and E. Zhirov, 1949 and by A. Bernstam, 1952.

    8. <u>Tshiung-Tipe</u> (Tshiung-Tepe) (in the Talas Valley). Ten intentionally formed skulls. Published by H. Heikel, 1918.

    9. <u>Bolsherechenskoe</u> Gorodishche (near Barnaul, West-Siberia). Published by E. Zhirov, 1940.

    10. <u>Kainsk</u> (Tomsk district). Published by E. Zhirov, 1940.

    11. <u>Chuvash</u> (near Tobolsk, on the River Irtis). One intentionally formed skull. Published by H. Heikel, 1894.

    12. <u>Ust-Tartash</u> (Barabinsk steppe). One intentionally formed skull. Published by G. Debetz, 1948.

    13. V. Ginzburg (1954) published several intentionally formed skulls from At-Bashi and Kzyl-Kyshtak from the first centuries B.C. and A.D., and from Kzyl-Tura and Kurgak from the 2nd-4th centuries A.D. All of the sites are in South Kirghizstan.

    14. <u>Blizhnye Elbany</u> (south of Barnaul at Bolshaya Rechka, on the right bank of the River Ob, in the northern part of Altai). Five intentionally formed skulls dating from between the 2nd century B.C. and 1st century A.D. have been excavated by the North-Altai expedition led by M. Griaznov in 1946-1949. Published by V. Alekseyev, 1956.

    15. Numerous intentionally formed skulls have been unearthed in the <u>Kurgans south of Isik-köl</u>, in the <u>Zalai Valley</u> on the right bank of the Kizik-Su River and in the <u>Minusinsk Basin</u>. Published by V. Ginzburg, 1950; mentioned by G. Debetz, 1948.

16. In several other parts of Central Asia intentionally formed skulls have been reported, e.g. Gur-Miron(Kazakh Republic) one skull; Vrevskaya railway station (one skull) V. Ginzburg, 1956); at Khoresm (L. Oshanin, 1953), Kuba-Tau (on the left bank of the River Khoresm) etc. Published by T. Trofimova, 1959.

The custom of head formation survived up to recent times in the Central Asian territories (for details see: Sovietskaya Etnografia, Moskva, VI-VII, and R. Basutti, 1967).

Intentionally formed skulls have also been found at Fergana from the 5th-3rd centuries B.C., in Turkmenistan from the 5th-4th centuries B.C. and in Central-Kazakhstan from the 3rd-1st centuries B.C.

2. **Finds from the Caspian Sea and along the River Dnieper**

   1. Brodi (Perm province, near Kungur). One skull. Published by E. Zhirov, 1940.
   2. Shardinsk. One skull. Published by E. Zhirov, 1940 (after Chugunov).
   3. Mias. Published by A. Heikel, 1894.
   4. Pershino (Cheliabinsk, on the bank of the River Mias). Published by K. Shalnikov, 1950.
   5. Kalmitzky Brod (Sverdlovsk). Published by K. Shalnikov, 1950.
   6. Agapovsk (12 kilometres south of Magnitogorsk). Published by K. Shalnikov, 1950.
   7. Djanatan (Orsk). Published by K. Shalnikov, 1940; E. Zhirov, 1940.
   8. Biis-Oba (on the River Berdianka, near Blagoslovensk at Chkalov-Orenburg). Published by B. Grakov, 1929; K. Smirnov, 1948.
   9. Nizhny Bashkunchak (Lake Bashkunchak, Astrakan district). Published by P. Rykov, 1928.
   10. Boaro (Kalmytzkaya Gora). Published by I. Sinitzyn, 1946.
   11. Elista (Kalmyk steppe). Published by P. Rykov, 1936.
   12. Abganer (Autonomous, Kalmuk Territory). Published by P. Rykov, 1929.
   13. Maly Useni River district. Published by P. Rao, 1926.
   14. Semiglavy Mar (Derkul, east of the Riazan-Uralsk railway, at Shipov). Published by P. Rykov, 1926 and T. Minaeva, 1927.
   15. Berezhniky (Buguruslan district, between Kuibishev and Samara). Several skulls. Published by A. Schmidt, 1926 and E. Zhirov, 1940.
   16. Kr. Yai (Kuibishev-Samara district). An extremely "deformed" skull. Published by D. Anuchin, 1887 and E. Dingwall, 1931.
   17. Susli (River Volga). Nine intentionally formed skulls from 53 kurgans. Published by P. Rykov, 1925.

18. Khutor Shulz (Torgan). Skulls from 4 kurgans. Published by P. Rao, 1927.

19. Engelsk-Petrovsk-Astrakhan (between the two settlements). Skulls from kurgans. Published by P. Rao, 1926.

20. Torgun. Skulls from three kurgans. Published by P. Rao, 1926.

21. Bangert (on the River Volga, south of Engelsk-Petrovsk). Published by P. Rao, 1926.

22. Gmelinskaya. Published by P. Rao, 1926.

23. Kharkovka (in the Köppen Valley). Published by P. Rao, 1926.

24. Kano (in the Köppen Valley). Published by P. Rao, 1926.

25. "Alt Weimar" (in: Werner, 1956). Its present name is unknown. Skulls from three kurgans. Published by P. Rao, 1927.

26. Karaman. Skulls from two kurgans. Published by P. Rao, 1927.

27. Atkarsk (north-west of Saratov). Skulls from two kurgans. Published by N. Artziutov.

28. Norka (south-west of Saratov). Published by P. Rao, 1926.

29. Chernokleevsk (2 kilometres east of Karpovka, along the Volgograd-Kalach railway). From two kurgans. Published by K. Smirnov, 1950.

30. Ilinka (on the River Sal, Don district). Extremely "deformed" skull, published by K. Zhaiuta, 1925.

31. Rostov-on-Don. One skull. Published by E. Dingwall, 1931.

32. Veseli (on the Manich Channel, Rostov district). Mentioned in Arkheologicheskie Isledovania v RSFSR, 1934-1936 (1941), p. 204.

33. Stanitza Melekhovskaya (Rostov district). Published by E. Zhirov, 1940.

34. Kobiakovo Gorodishche (Abaisk, Rostov district). Published by E. Zhirov, 1940.

35. Taganrog. Published by E. Zhirov, 1940.

36. Nieshcheretovo-Nieshcherove (Voroshilovgrad district, Belokurakinsk province. Finds from two kurgans. Published by I. Lutzkevich, 1952.

37. Vorontzovka (Kupiansk district, on the River Senikha). Published by E. Melnik, 1902.

38. Novo-Filipovka (Molochnaya, north-east of Melitopol). Published by M. Viasmitina, 1953, and P. Efimenko and I. Shovkoplias, 1954.

39. Bogodar (Aleksandrovsk district, earlier Ekaterinoslav province). Published by P. Rao, 1926 and E. Zhirov, 1940.

40. Emchikha (Kaniev district). Published by N. Brandenburg, 1889.

41. Cherniakhov (Kiev district). One intentionally formed skull from a large cemetery with 251 graves. Published by B. Khvoiko, 1901 and J. Kukharenko, 1954.

42. Krasnogorka (Tirapol district). Published by E. Zhirov, 1940.

43. Belbek (Crimea, north of Sevastopol). Published by G. Moiberg, 1946.

44. Berezhnovka and Kalinovka (near Volgagrad). 43 intentionally formed skulls have been found, 28 of men, 15 of women. Published by B. Firstein, 1970.

3. Finds from the Caucasus

1. Some skulls have been found at Gurzuf and Gugush from the 10th century B.C. (A. Kharuzin), and 19 skulls have been found at Nalchik, near Ordzhonikidze, from the 12th-11th centuries B.C. by G. Vertepov. They were published partly by H. Field (1953) and partly by R. Martin. The skulls were considerably formed by circular bandages. 16 skulls belonged to men, 3 to women.

2. Phanagoria (on the Taman Peninsula). Out of the 18 graves of the cemetery contained intentionally formed skulls. Published by V. Blavatzky, 1951.

3. Borishovo (Novorossiisk). From the part of the cemetery used in its first period, two intentionally formed skulls have been reported. Published by E. Zhirov, 1940, in Izvestia Imperatorskoy Arkheologicheskoy Komissii, LVI, (1914), p. 84.

4. Pashkova Stanitza (18 kilometres from Krasnodar). Two intentionally formed skulls have been excavated in cemeteries nos. I and III. Published by K. Smirnov, 1951.

5. Giliach (on the upper River Kuban). 17 skulls. Published by T. Minaeva, 1951.

6. Oshokurova (Urushbevo) (Upper Bakshan, Piatigorska district). 12 skulls. Published by E. Chantre, 1887; V. Miller, 1888; R. Virchow, 1888; E. Dingwall, 1931 and E. Zhirov, 1940.

7. Otluk-Kala (on the River Grundelen, Upper-Bakshan). At least one skull. Published by E. Chantre, 1887; E. Dingwall, 1931 (?) and E. Zhirov, 1940.

8. Giigit (on the left bank of the upper River Bakshan). Numerous intentionally formed skulls, published by T. Minaeva, 1951.

9. Kurkushan (Nalchik district). Several intentionally formed skulls. Published by E. Zhirov, 1940 and mentioned in Eurasia Septentrionalis Antiqua, Helsinki, V (1930), p. 216.

10. Baital-Chapkan (south of Stavropol). Several skulls. Published by T. Minaeva, 1951.

11. On the River Mara (tributary of the Kukan). Numerous skulls. Published by T. Minaeva, 1951.

12. Zadalisk (Urus). 8 intentionally formed skulls. Published by E. Zhirov, mentioned in Materiali po Arkheologii Kavkaza, VIII (1900), pp. 191 and 195.

13. Chegem (Piatigorsk district). Several skulls. Published by P. Rao, 1926; Eberts Reallexikon d. Vorgeschichte XIII (1929), p. 109; in Materiali po Arkheologii Kavkaza I (1888).

14. Kamunta (on the River Sugunta, at Urush). Several finds, published by P. Rao, 1926; Eberts Reallexikon d. Vorgeschichte XIII (1929), p. 109; Materiali po Arkheologii Kavkaza VIII (1900), p. 293 ff.

15. Georgievsk (on the left bank of the Upper Kuban River). A double grave of a man and a woman. Mentioned in Materiali po Arkheologii Kavkaza IX (1904), p. 145ff.

16. Vladikavkaz. Several finds. Published by P. Rao, 1926 p. 107 and also in Eberts Reallexikon d. Vorgeschichte XIII (1929), p. 109.

17. Mozdok (near Vladikavkaz). One intentionally formed skull. Published by E. Zhrivov, 1940; mentioned in Ar'kheologicheskie Issledovania v RSFSR 1934-1936 (1941), p. 240.

18. Mishatzkaya Stanitza (on the River Terek). One intentionally formed skull. Published by P. Uvarova, 1902.

19. Prokhladnaya Stanitza (on the River Terek). Two intentionally formed skulls. Published by P. Uvarova, 1902.

20. Alkhan-Kala (Chechen-Ingush Autonomous SSR). Published by E. Zhirov, 1940.

21. Tiemir-Khan-Shura (Dagestan). Several intentionally formed skulls. Published by A. Zakharov, 1930 and B. Posta, 1905.

22. Djemi-Kent (Dagestan). One skull. Published by E. Zhirov, 1940.

23. Samtavro (at Tbilisi). 26 intentionally formed skulls. Published by E. Chantre, 1886; E. Dingwall, 1931; E. Zhirov, 1940 and mentioned in Zeitschrift für Ethnologie IV (1872), p. 12.

24. Mtzkhet (Tbilisi). Three skulls. Published by E. Zhirov, 1940, and V. Ginzburg and E. Zhirov, 1949.

25. Cheremi (50 kilometres from Signakh). Published by E. Zhirov, 1940.

26. Sartachali. Published by E. Dingwall, 1931 and E. Zhirov, 1940.

The custom of intentional head formation has survived for a long time and is still customary among the Osets and the Katvelies, so this custom cannot be ascribed to peoples arriving from outside, but is an ancient tradition among the aboriginals of the Caucasus who acquired this custom, in all probability, from peoples living in Iran. In more recent times comparative examinations have been carried out among peoples in this region practising the custom of head formation and those leaving the heads of the infants in the original form. V. Miller's (1881-1887), A. Ivanovski's (1891), N. Gilchenko's (1890) and later M. Levin's (1947) examinations led to interesting results. The head-index (Martin 8:1 measurement) in cases of slight formation was 76.3, in cases of medium strong formation was 75.4, and in cases of extreme formation was 74.4 instead of the standard of 78.9. The findings indicate the continuity of the practice.

4. Finds from South Russia, the Ukraine and the Crimea

   1. Shipovo (on the River Derkul, along the Riazan-Uralsk railway). Two intentionally formed skulls, published by T. Mianeva—V. Mashlovsky, 1929 and E. Zhirov, 1940.

   2. Ufa (Ulitza Karl Marx). Published by R. Akhmerov, 1951.

   3. Ufa (Ulitza Sotzialista). Published by R. Akhmerov, 1951.

   4. Engels-Petrovsk (Voskhod). One fragmentary skull. Published by I. Sinitzin, 1936.

   5. Engels-Petrovsk (3-4 kilometres south-east of the town). Published by I. Sinitzin, 1936.

   6. Ilovatki (Volgograd district). Published by K. Smirnov, 1953.

   7. Morsker Chulek (at Nedvigorsky Gorodishche). Published by E. Zhirov, 1940.

   8. Cherenki (Dniepropetrovsk). Published by E. Zhirov, 1940.

   9. Olbia. Two extremely formed skulls. Published by E. Zhirov, 1940.

   10. Khersonessos (Crimea). 39 intentionally formed skulls. Mentioned in Otchet Imperatorskoy Arkheologicheskoy Komissii I (1893), p. 73; Izvestia Impertorskoy Arkheologicheskoy Komissii XXV (1907), pp. 74, 126; Materiali i Issledovania po Arkheologii SSSR XXXIV (1953), p. 253; E. Dingwall, 1931; V. Ginzburg and E. Zhirov, 1949.

   11. Kerch (Crimea). One skull was sent to Prof. Bauermeister to Köln in 1953, another one was found in the catacombs on Mithriades Hill. The latter is mentioned in Izvestia Imperatorskoy Arkheologicheskoy Komissii XXX, p. 30; V. Ginzburg and E. Zhirov, 1949. Apart from these two skulls, 34 intentionally formed skulls are mentioned from Kertch.

   12. Suuk-Su (Yalta). In the 93 graves of a Gothic cemetery 11 intentionally formed skulls were found. Published by N. Repnikov, 1906.

   13. Alushta (Crimea). 11 intentionally formed skulls. Published by V. Ginzburg and E. Zhirov, 1949.

   14. Gurzuf (near Yalta). Several intentionally formed skulls. Mentioned in Izvestia Imperatorskoy Arkheologicheskoy Komissii XIX (1906), p. 33.

   15. Eshki Kermen (Crimea). 3 skulls. Published by N. Repnikov, 1932.

   16. Inkerman (Crimea). Mentioned in Izvestia Imperatorskoy Arkheologicheskoy Kommissii XX (1906), p. 33; E. Dingwall, 1931.

17. Bia-Salie (Crimea). Mentioned in Izvestia Imperatorskoy Arkheologicheskoy Komissii XIX (1906), p. 33; E. Dingwall, 1931.

The intentionally formed skulls of our era (the Sarmatian period, the time of Attila, etc.) can be traced back to earlier periods and originate in regions to the south or south-east. The greatest complex of such finds is the Kenkol group, reminiscent of western Alan and western Hun finds, which allow us to draw the conclusion that the custom of head formation was first used by the Huns living in Kangkü under some degree of Iranian influence. The origin is therefore to be sought among the Iranians. Intentional head formation was not practised in south Siberia (Minusisnk Basin) until the first centuries A.D., when some groups in the Tienshan (Talas Valley), at Isik-köl and in the Pamir (Alai Valley) suddenly took over the custom.

The "Huns" of the Kenkol group have nothing to do ethnically with the Central Asian, south Siberian, Tunguz-Mandzhu, north Chinese or Tibetian mongoloids according to V. Ginzburg and E. Zhirov. They try to ascribe the group and also the custom to the South Turkestanian Uigurs. K. Smirnov (1950) attributes the custom to the Ukranian Kushnans, occupying Baktiria and North India at the beginning of our era. J. Werner (1956), in his paper which is full of contradictions, writes (p. 11);

> "die Schädelform in Mittelasien auf die mongolische Kenkol-Gruppe im Tiensan und Pamir beschränkt ist und es eine Zukunftsaufgabe der Forschung sein wird, mit der Herkunft der Kenkol-Gruppe auch die Herkunft der mit ihr so eng verknüpften Schädelbildung zu klären...."

Later in the same paper, dealing with the head formation of the Sarmations he writes:

> "die Sitte der Schädelformation kam aus dem Osten zu den Sarmaten".

Later he called this eastern people 'Huns'. Such finds in South Russia can be ascribed to the Sarmatians, to the Goths living in the Crimea on the Black Sea, and other Germanic peoples. The Hun invasion drove many peoples into Europe, some of them being absorbed in the mass of people called "Huns", some of them going on westwards. Such were the Alans of Iranian origin, the Germanic Goths, the Gepids and the Sarmatians living in great numbers in the South Russian steppe region.

The scope of this paper does not allow us to discuss the biological changes of the crania in the course of formation, a study of which was carried out by H. Helmuth in 1970. However, it must be mentioned. When identifying the peoples arriving from the east in central Europe in our era, most of the misinterpretations are due to a lack of understanding of these changes. The strong encircling bandages pressing on the forehead makes the root of the nose flatter and wider, the face more prognathous, the zygomatic processes are made more outstanding at the sides, and the whole head gives "mongoloid" impression. After a realistic re-examination of the finds, many mongoloid skulls proved to belong to peoples using and spreading the custom of head formation in Eurasia. Maybe this misinterpretation was partly responsible for the fact that the Huns were considered for a long time to be mongoloid. Mongoloid characteristics are hardly if ever detectable among the South Russian finds.

INTENTIONALLY FORMED SKULLS IN SOUTH AND SOUTH-EAST EUROPE (ROMANIA, BULGARIA, GREECE, JUGOSLAVIA AND ITALY)

ROMANIA

1. **Constanta.** 4 intentionally formed skulls have been discovered together with 60 skulls of normal form. Published by E. Pittard, 1900-1901.

2. **Trusesti** (near Jijia). Mentioned in Studi si cercetari ist. veche, Bucharest, III (1952), pp. 83, 117.

3. **Vadului-Voda** (Bessarabia). Published by A. Donici, 1931.

4. **Pogorasti** (Botosani district, Suceava). 4 skeletons have been excavated, the second of which (archaeologically defined as Sarmatian dating back to the 3rd century A.D.) had an intentionally formed skull. The skull of a man was medium formed. Published by M. Critescu, 1964.

5. **Tirgsor.** Diaconu (1965) published both archaeological and anthropological finds from cemeteries from the 3rd-4th century A.D. In the first cemetery, archaeologically dating from the 3rd century A.D., 10 skulls out of 20 (possibly Sarmatians) were intentionally formed. Detailed anthropological evaluation is still awaited. As well as Diaconu (1965), S. Nicolaescu-Plopsor has worked on the finds.

6. **Tatina** (near Spantov). The skull of a 60 year old man. Published by O. Necrasov and S. Antoniu, 1962.

BULGARIA

1. **Novi Pasar.** The Bulgarian Academy of Sciences carried out archaeological excavations on the site in 1948-1949. Among the skeletons excavated (Protobulgarians from the 8th-9th century A.D.) two had intentionally formed skulls. One of them belonged to an old man (grave 19) the other to a younger woman (grave 28). Published by P. Boev, 1957.

GREECE

No skulls with intentional head formation dating from historical times have been found in Greece. Those excavated in Cyprus have already been mentioned in the chapter dealing with the custom of head formation. An extremely "deformed" skull was found about a hundred years ago at Trikeri (Volos-Thessaly) but neither its origin nor its ethnic place are known. The find is not yet published, but can be found in the Athens Anthropological Museum under inventory number Tv 7 (information from N. Xirotiris).

JUGOSLAVIA

1. **Jakovo** (Surcin, in Slavonia). Intentionally formed skulls were found in the 19 graves of a cemetery dating from the 6th century A.D. Anthropological examinations have not yet been carried out. Mentioned by V. Lebzelter in Forschung und Forschritte XI (1935), p.319.

2. S. Kanzian (on the Istrian Peninsula). In Tominz cave a skeleton was uncovered 50 centimetres below a Roman grave in 1894. The skeleton had no grave goods. Published by R. Battaglia, 1942.

3. Kranj (in Slovenia, on the Sava River). Th. Pavslar, J. Szombathy, J. Zmauc and W. Schmid excavated 650 graves from the 5th-6th centuries in 1898 and 1905. One part of the cemetery was used by the Ostrogoths, another by the Langobards, while the people buried here were mainly local inhabitants. 73 of the skeletons were transferred to the Anthropologische Abteilung of the Vienna Naturhistorisches Museum, labelled "Grabung Szombathy, 1901, 1902". The bone material from the cemetery was identified and published after the Second World War by I. Kiszely in 1970. The skulls of three old women were intentionally formed; very probably they were found in the Ostrogothic part of the cemetery.

4. Rakovcani (Prijedora, Bosnia). N. Miletic excavated a cemetery dating from the 5th-6th centuries in 1960-1964. Out of the 66 graves in the cemetery, 3 men and a woman had intentionally formed skulls. The anthropological examination was carried out by G. Pilaric in 1970.

5. Dravlje (Ulica Gotska, Ljubljana, Slovenia). M. Slaba excavated in 1968 59 graves from a cemetery belonging partly to the Goths. The examination of the intentionally formed skulls was begun by T. Pogacnik, but his sudden death delayed its completion. A preliminary publication of the finds was made by M. Slabe. He also published in 1970-1971 another extremely formed skull from grave 19.

6. Rifnik (12 kilometres east of Celje). On a hill at Celje a cemetery with 93 graves from the 2nd-4th centuries was excavated in the vicinity of an Illyrian urn grave. The director of the excavations was L. Bolta (1968). He wrote during the analysis of the material: "Bei einen Skelette (grave no. 56) konnte man unverkennbare zeichnen einen absichtlichen Deformation des Schädels bemerken". He also published a photograph of the skull. T. Pognacnik later took over the study of the material, and after his death other experts continued the work, which is still in hand.

7. Ptuj (c. 25 kilometres south-east of Maribor). The extremely formed skull of a man was unearthed from beneath the Prostipska Church in Ptuj in 1973. The find has been deposited in the Museum with the inventory number 13539. The finds are being analysed by J. Hadzsi.

8. Bled. B. Skerlj mentioned an intentionally formed skull from grave 226 of the cemetery excavated at Bled. He published its anthropological data in 1953.

ITALY

1. Padova (Piazza Capitaniato). The skull of a woman was found in the last century (perhaps in the 1870s). Probably it can be ascribed to the Goths. Published by G. Ganestrini and L. Moschen, 1878, and later in detail by P. Bellasi, 1962.

2. Casalechio (6 kilometres from Bologna). The intentionally formed skull of an old man was first published by G. Sergi (1890) and later in detail by E. Dingwall (1931) and P. Belassi (1962).

3. Fusco (Siracusa). The skull found by Orsi in 1893 has been mentioned several times. It was published at last by P. Bellasi in 1962.

4. Isnello (near Palermo). The slightly or medium formed head of a woman was found in a cave in 1906. It was first published by V. Giuffrida-Ruggieri in 1906 and later in detail by P. Bellasi in 1962.

5. Fiesole (Firenze). First two (1873), and later (1909-1910) several more skeletons dating from the Early Migration Period have been unearthed in Piazza Umberto I (now Piazza Mino). Archaeologically the finds were ascribed to the "Langobards" while anthropologically they belonged to the "Goths". The 2nd grave contained the skeleton of a 30 year old woman, whose head had undergone rather considerable intentional formation in infancy. The finds were published by I. Kiszely in 1970.

6. Gaudo. Several intentionally formed skulls have been found in Italy from the Prehistoric times. The greatest number came from Gaudo and date from 2,000 B.C. The publication and the analysis of the finds in 1970 are still going on. The material is in the Instituto di Antropologia at Pisa. The examination is being carried out by F. Mallegni.

INTENTIONALLY FORMED SKULLS FOUND IN THE CARPATHIAN BASIN REGION

1. Székelyudvarhely (Transylvania). The intentionally formed skull found in 1874 was the second find in its kind in Hungary. It was first described by M. Steiburg in 1875, and was published by J. Lenhossék in 1878.

2. Szászbonyha (Transylvania). An intentionally formed skull was found in 1899. Published by L. Bartucz, 1938.

3. Arad-Gáj (Transylvania). 5 intentionally formed skulls were found in a large cemetery ascribed to the Gepids in 1897 and 1903. L. Bartucz described them first in Szegedi Dolgozatok XII (1936), p. 28, and later in 1938.

4. Elek (near Arad). Two intentionally formed skulls were found in a cemetery ascribed to the Gepids in 1927 and 1929. Published by L. Bartucz, 1938.

5. Pancsevo (Pancevo) (Banat, now in Jugoslavia). Three intentionally formed skulls were excavated in 1879 and 1883. Published by J. Lenhossék, 1886, and L. Bartucz, 1938.

6. Vinkovci (Banat). Two intentionally formed skulls were excavated in 1908. Published by L. Bartucz, 1938.

7. Subotica (Szabadka Sándor Co-operative, Bánat). An extremely formed skull of a woman was found in 1950. Published by Gy. Farkas, 1973.

8. Subotica (Szabadka)—Huszárkaszárnya (Bácska). The badly preserved skull of a child was found in 1963. Published by Gy. Farkas, 1973.

9. Ada (Bácska). An extremely formed skull of a man was found, and is now in the Novi Sad Museum. Published by Gy. Farkas, 1973.

10. Tápé-Lebősziget (Szeged). The intentionally formed skull of a woman was found in the part of the cemetery ascribed to the Gepids by the archaeologists. Published by Gy. Farkas and P. Lipták, 1971.

11. Szekszárd (Tolna). The intentionally formed skull of a 40-50 year old man. Published by L. Bartucz, 1938.

12. Dombovár (Tolna). An intentionally formed skull was found in 1883. Archaeologically it is dated to the 5th century. Published by L. Bartucz, 1938.

13. Csongrád-Tiszapart (c. Csongrád). This intentionally formed skull was the first of its kind found in Hungary. It was published by J. Lenhossék in 1878 and L. Bartucz in 1938. Another intentionally formed skull was found in 1935 (Bartucz, 1938) at a site called "Csongrád-városháza" should be mentioned.

14. Bátaszék (Tolna). An intentionally formed skull was found in 1890. Published by L. Bartucz, 1938.

15. Szeged. Two intentionally formed skulls. Published by L. Bartucz, 1938.

16. Velemszentvid (c. Vas). The intentionally formed skulls of a woman and a child were found. Mentioned by R. Virchow, 1890; later in Mitt. des Anthrop. Ges. in Wien XXXIII (1903), p. 33; then published by A. Török (1904), A. Schitz (1905) and L. Bartucz, 1938.

17. Lengyel (Tolna). An intentionally formed skull of a woman dating from the Bronze Age. Virchow found it worthy of detailed consideration. He noticed that the skeleton was buried in a contracted position, thus differing from burials of the Migration Period. Published by R. Virchow, 1890; A. Schlitz, 1905, and L. Bartucz, 1938.

18. Ószőny (the Roman Brigetio; c. Komárom). The intentionally formed skull of a man was found in the Roman castrum. Published by J. Lenhossék, 1884, 1886; A. Schliz, 1905; L. Bartucz, 1938.

19. Gyöngyösapáti-Kápolnadomb (now Gencsapáti; c. Vas). The intentionally formed skull of a 20 year old man was found in 1941. Published by J. Nemeskéri, 1944-1945.

20. Szirmabesenyő-Szirmateseny (c. Borsod-Abauj-Zemplén). The skull of a man was found in 1950, and is now in the Miskolc Museum. Published by G. Megay, 1952 and J. Nemeskéri, 1952.

21. Győr (The library of the Benedictine Abbey). The skull of a 20-24

year old man was excavated in the vicinity of Győr during E. Lovas's excavations in 1950. Published by J. Nemeskéri, 1952.

22. Győr-Széchenyi Square. The skull of a child (Infant II) was found in 1959 during A. Uzsoki's excavation in the Late Roman cemetery. Published by J. Nemeskéri, 1952.

23. Mohács (c. Baranya). The skull of a 30-35 year old man was discovered during the excavations at Mohács in 1949 financed by the Hungarian National Museum. Published by J. Nemeskéri, 1952.

24. Keszthely-Fenékpuszta (The northern shore of Lake Balaton, C. Veszprém). A fragmentary skull of an 8-9 year old child was found in grave 35, ascribed to the Huns. Published by J. Nemeskéri, 1952.

Later, during the Soviet-Hungarian joint excavations in 1976-1977 ten graves were unearthed in the Gothic part of the cemetery, 9 of which contained skeletons with intentionally formed skulls. The finds will be examined by I. P Papp, of the Hungarian Museum of Natural Science. The excavation is to be continued in 1978.

25. Adony (C. Fejér). The intentionally formed skull of a c. 2 year old child was found during the excavations carried out by the Hungarian National Museum in 1949. The skeleton was lying in the Late Roman part of the cemetery. Published by J. Nemeskéri, 1952.

26. Domolospuszta (Zsibót) (Szigetvár, C. Baranya). An intentionally formed skull was found in the 1950s by J. Dombay, Director of the Janus Pannonius Museum at Pécs. The find was published by Gy. Regöly-Merei (1962) from the medical historical and pathological point of view.

27. Gyula (C. Békés). Four intentionally formed skulls were found in a cemetery ascribed by the archaeologists to the Gepids. Three intentionally formed skulls were found at Gyula-Kálvária dűlő in 1901-1902 and one at Gyula-Kétegyháza Road in 1928. Published by L. Bartucz, 1938.

28. Szentes (C. Csongrád). Two intentionally formed skulls were found in 1895 in a cemetery ascribed by the archaeologists to the Gepids. Published by L. Bartucz, 1938. The archaeological excavations and finds were published and described by D. Csallány in A Szegedi Városi Muzeum Kiadványai (Publications of the Szeged Municipal Museum) II, 4 (1943), p. 35.

29. Hódmezővásárhely (Gorzsa tanya) (C. Csongrád). The grave no. 93 in the Gepid cemetery contained the intentionally formed skull of a woman. The finds were published by G. Gáspár in 1931 and 1933. The archaeological finds were published by J. Banner in 1931 in Szegedi Dolgozatok.

30. Kiszombor (near Szeged, C. Csongrád). F. Móra has excavated 426 graves from a Gepid cemetery. 63 graves contained anthropologically determinable skulls, 21 of which were intentionally formed. 19 belonged to men, two to women. Published by L. Bartucz, 1938 and 1966.

31. Szőreg-Téglagyár (Brickfabric) (a part of Szeged from 1973). L. Bartucz (1966) described 9 intentionally formed skulls from the Gepid cemetery excavated in 1927-1929. 5 of them belonged to men, 4 to women. The numbers of the graves containing the intentionally formed skulls were: 10, 11, 47, 75, 85, 89, 91b, 124 and 126. No detailed publication is available.

32. Tököl (near Budapest, on Csepel Island, C. Pest). A find which presents many problems. An intentionally formed skull together with the skeleton was found in a Bronze Age cemetery. L. Bartucz wrote of it (1938): "grave No. 23 contained the skeleton of a 35-40 year old man. No doubt it was buried in a contracted position. A bronze hair-ring was lying by the left temple." It is also notable that the skull was called "macrocephalic" (p. 12). From the authentic drawing and photograph of the grave, L. Bartucz states that "as the cemetery undoubtedly dates from the beginning of the Bronze Age and as the skeleton was lying in an undisturbed grave in the cemetery, the custom of intentional head formation was already practised at the beginning of the Bronze Age in our country, not as general custom but as a privilege of certain families (p. 16). The excavation of the cemetery was carried out in 1913.

Another extremely formed skull, mentioned by L. Bartucz in 1938, was found in grave No. 113 of the cemetery.

33. Hács-Béndekpuszta (C. Somogy). I. Pusztai during rescur excavations in 1954 excavated 25 graves from the Germanic Period. The grave No. 23 contained the extremely formed skull of a woman. Published by P. Lipták, 1961, and I. Kiszely, 1973.

34. Sövényháza (C. Csongrád). A skull was found in 1903. Published by L. Bartucz, 1938.

35. Kesztölc (near Esztergom, C. Komárom). The extremely formed skull of a 16-17 year old man has been found at house No. 11, Petőfi Street, in 1963. Published by I. Kiszely, 1972.

36. Soponya (C. Fejér). A Marosi excavated a grave with rich grave-goods in 1936 and later I. Bóna during verifying excavations in 1959 found the last three graves of the cemetery. The skull found in 1936 has been lost, but all the three graves unearthed by I. Bóna contained skeletons with intentionally formed skulls. In grave No. 2 was a 17 year old woman, in the No. 3 a 40 year old woman and in No. 4 an 18-20 year old man. Published by I. Kiszely, 1976.

37. Tamási-Adorjánpuszta (C. Tolna). During the excavation of the foundations of a building in the Uj Élet Co-operative the extremely formed skull and the skeleton of a 30-35 year old man dating from the Early Migration Period was found. Published by I. Hankó and I. Kiszely, 1971-1972.

38. Letkés (C. Nógrád). L. Papp excavated 3 graves from the Early Migration Period in 1965. They are likely to belong to the Quadi population. A woman, a child and a man were lying in the graves, and all had intentionally formed skulls. Published by I. Kiszely, 1971.

39. Regöly (C. Tolna). A rich grave from the Early Migration Period was found in 1967 in a sandpit. The grave contained the intentionally formed skull of a c. 35 year old woman. Published by I. Hankó, 1968.

In the last few years more and more intentionally formed skulls have been discovered in the Carpathian Basin, the anthropological analyses of which have not yet been carried out. They are as follows:

40. Mosonszentjános—Hansági tanyák (Hanság settlement) (C. Győr-Sopron). Excavations by Gy. Pusztai, 1961.

41. Tatabánya (C. Komárom)

42. Győr-Kálváriadomb. Four intentionally formed skulls.

43. Tiszavasvári-Paptelekhát (C. Szabolcs-Szatmár)

44. Tiszadob-Sziget (C. Szabolcs-Szatmár). D. Csallány directed excavations in 1957 in a Sarmatian cemetery from the Hun period. Two intentionally formed skulls were found.

45. Szabolcs-Calvinist vicarage (C. Szabolcs-Szatmár). In a robbed grave (No. 18) of the cemetery the intentionally formed skull of a young person was found in 1977. The find will be examined and published by L. Szathmáry.

46. Szőny-Téglagyár (Brick factory) (C. Komárom). 6 intentionally formed skulls have been discovered.

47. Szolnok-Szanda, repülőter (airport). Gy. Kaposvári directed the excavations of a Gepid cemetery.

48. Mőzs (C. Tolna). Several intentionally formed skulls were found in 1961 during the excavations directed by Á. Salamon.

49. Szekszárd-Palánk (C. Tolna). Three intentionally formed skulls were discovered during the excavations directed by Á. Salamon in 1959.

50. Vác (C. Pest). A longitudinally formed skull was found in the sand-pit.

51. Kunaolacs-Alsóadacs (C. Bács-Kiskun). Petőfi Street.

52. Baja (C. Bács-Kiskun).

53. Pilismarót (C. Komárom)

54. Hird (C. Baranya). An intentionally formed skull was excavated in a great cemetery from the Migration Period in 1967. The excavations were directed by V. Kováts.

55. Szanda-Szőlőkaljapuszta (C. Nógrád)

56. Szentes (C. Csongrád). Intentionally formed skulls have been found at Nagyhegy, Nagytőke, Berekhát and Kökényzug in Gepid cemeteries excavated by G. Csallány.

57. Madaras-Halmok (C. Bács-Kiskun). An intentionally formed skull was found in a great cemetery from the Sarmatian-Hun period, during M. Kőhegyi's excavations in 1968.

58. Dunaújváros (the Roman Intercisa). The cemetery of the Roman settlement dating from the 2nd-3rd centuries A.D. has been excavated over many years. The number of graves excavated has increased between 1964 and 1976 from 86 to 2217, and the excavations are still going on. The anthropological and archaeological examinations are also continuing. The analyses of the human bones is carried out by I. Kiszely. The inhabitants of the trading centre and legionary fort excavated by E. Vágó and Zs. Visy consisted of the local population, Italian Romans and the south-eastern Asian cohort of archers. After the Romans were driven from Pannonia the territory was peopled by Germanic tribes.

In the part of the cemetery studied in detail so far 9 skeletons have been found with intentionally formed skulls: graves 31 (50 year old man), 40 (adult to senile man), 79 (adult woman), 210 (adult man), 402 (probably a woman), 600 (probably a man), 1481 (30 year old woman), 1485 (50-55 year old man), 1492 (35 year old woman).

As only a half of the cemetery has been studied in detail it is highly probable that more intentionally formed skulls will be found later. The skeletons with formed heads make up a coherent part of the cemetery proving that the local population remained in Intercisa after the Romans' departure, and were absorbed into the groups of new-comers.

59. Rácalmás-Rózsamajor (C. Fejér). 157 Avar graves dating from the 7th century have been excavated by I. Bóna and Zs. Visy in 1971. In grave no. 113 the skull of a 50 year-old woman was intentionally formed. Neither the archaeological finds nor the human bones have been published.

The skull is medium formed. Its anthropological characteristics: brachycranial, hypsicranic, metriocranic, medium narrow forehead, metrio-eurymetopic, orthognathous, mesorene, mesoconchic, leptostaphyline. The form of the skull is sphaenoides. Phaenoprosopic, phaenozygia, medium large tubera parietalia, medium large glabella, large processus mastoideus (especially for a woman), medium wide apertura piriformis, medium deep fossa canina, narrow porus acusticus slanting forwards, the zygomatic processes stand out on the sides, the zygomatics are narrow, the palate is shoe-formed and low, foramen occipitale magnum is oval narrowing backwards, one os suturarum on the left side. Caries media on the upper 7th tooth on the left side. Mesodontes.

The formation of the head was carried out with circular bandages.

60. Fertőszentimiklós-Szereti dűlő (C. Győr-Sopron). Several intentionally formed skulls have been unearthed in 1971 in a cemetery with archaeological finds from the Germanic Period. One of the skulls was sent to Csorna Local History Museum where it can be found today. The archaeological excavations were directed by P. Tomka, an archaeologist from Győr, but no more intentionally formed skulls were found. The skull, without the jaw, belonged to a 25 year old man. Its anthropological characteristics: mesocranial, ortho-hypsicranial, metriocranic, narrow forehead, stenometopic, mesognathous, mesorene, mesoconchic, leptorrhine, leptostaphyline, dolichuranic. The cranial bones are thick,

the form of the skull is ovoidal. Phaenoprosopic, phaenozygia, large tubera frontalia, small tubera parietalia, fundamental processus ossis, medium large processus mastoideus. The orbits are high and of rounded rectangular form, the nasal bone is medium large. The apertura piriformis is symmetrically medium wide, the zygomatic processes stand out on the sides. The palate is U-formed and medium high, foramen occipitale magnum is rounded. Mesodontes. Sutura metopica is present as in most cases of intentionally formed skulls. The head formation is considerable and was probably carried out with circular bandages.

61. <u>Csongrád-Bökény</u> (formerly Bökény-Mindszent, C. Csongrád). Germanic archaeological finds were reported and were deposited in the Szentes Museum as early as 1885. K. Nagy and M. Nagy have excavated, among others, 14 graves in 1971 (graves nos. 11-24), 3 of which contained intentionally formed skulls. The bones are badly preserved and the facial parts are usually missing.

<u>Grave No. 11</u>. The calotte, jaw and skeletal bones of a 30-40 year old man (?). Anthropological characteristics: brachycranial, hypsicranial, metriocranic, the form of the skull is rhomboidal. Large tubera parietalia, the occipital, due to the slight formation with bandages, is planoccipital. The margins of the orbits are medium thick, the processus mastoideus is medium large.

<u>Grave No. 15</u>. The calotte, jaw and skeletal bones of a 50 year old woman (?). Anthropological characteristics of the skull: dolichomesocranial, its form is ovoidal, the porus acusticus is narrow, slanting forwards. Protuberantia occipitalis externa, against the intentional head formation, is large, the formation is of small extent.

<u>Grave No. 17</u>. Calotte and skeletal bones of a 50-60 year old man. The skull suffered slight intentional formation. Anthropological characteristics: mesocranial, hypsicranial, metrio-macrocranic, metriometopic, orthognathous, mesoprosopic, leptorene, mesoconchic. The form of the skull is birsoides. Kryptoprosopic, phaenozygia, small tubera parietalia, planoccipital, high rectangular orbits. The fossa canina is medium deep, the zygomatic processes stand out slightly on the sides, the genial process is low pyramid, ossa in sutura sagittalis.

63. <u>Hódmezővásárhely-Gorzsa</u> (formerly Kishomok, C. Csongrád). F. Móra has excavated several graves from a large Gepid cemetery at the beginning of the century. Excavations were also carried out by I. Bóna in 1966-1968, who excavated graves nos. 24-105. The anthropological finds were sent to the Anthropological Institute of the József Attila University of Sciences at Szeged. In graves nos. 96 and 104 the skulls were intentionally formed. The first one belonged to a 50 year old man, the other to a 35 year old man. Both were formed with encircling bandages. The anthropological study has been carried out by I. Kiszely.

64. <u>Straže</u> (near Piestan). J. Neústupný and J. Malý reported about 3 graves unearthed between 1930 and 1935. That labelled II is now in Piestan Museum. It belonged to a 7-8 year old child whose head had been intentionally formed. Published by J. Malý in 1936 and E. Vlček in 1957.

65. <u>Kapusany</u> (Presov district). V. Budinský-Kricka has excavated graves from the Migration Period in 1939. The skull of a child found in grave 4/39 was intentionally formed. Published by E. Vlcek, 1956.

66. <u>Sarovce</u> (East of Nitra). An intentionally formed skull was found in a grave dating from the Migration Period. Published by E. Vlcek, 1957.

67. <u>Steinbrunn</u> (formerly Stinkenbrunn; Burgenland, Eisenstadt district). Several graves dating from the Migration Period were discovered during earth-moving work in 1949. The archaeological examination of the material found in 23 graves was carried out by H. Mitscha-Märheim in 1953 and 1966, while anthropological examinations were carried out by I. Kiszely in the Anthropologische Abteilung of the Vienna Naturhistorisches Museum in 1976. The skulls from graves nos. 3a, 16 and 17 were intentionally formed and similar characteristics can perhaps be seen on skulls from graves nos. 5, 14 and 23. Unfortunately, the bones are badly preserved and their evaluation is of rather dubious value. All the formed skulls belonged to women.

<u>Grave No. 3a</u>. The skeleton of a 35 year old woman. Her head was formed with double bandages. Anthropological characteristics of the skull: mesocranial, hypsicranial, metriocranic, steno-eurymetopic, mesorene-leptorene, mesoconchic, platyrrhine, leptostaphyline, brachyuranic, mesognathous. The form of the skull is ovoidal. Kryptoprosopic, kryptozygia, planooccipitalis, narrow sutura sphaenoparietalis, small tubera parietalia, 5 ossa suturarum on the right side and 4 on the left. Subrectnagular orbits, apertura piriformis is wide below, slight sulcus praenasalis, filled fossa canina. Occlusion: labidont. The jaw is missing.

<u>Grave No. 16</u>. The skeleton of a 50 year old woman. The skeletal bones are well preserved but the skull is represented only by the frontal part of the calotte and some fragments. It bears signs of intentional formation with double bandages. Anthropological characteristics: mesocranial, hypsicranial, metriocranic. The form of the skull is ovoidal-rhomboidal. Planooccipital, small tubera parietalia, also small processus mastoideus.

<u>Grave No. 17</u>. Well preserved calotte, fragmentary facial part and also fragmentary lower jaw of a 50 year old woman. The signs of osteoporosis generans are clearly visible. Anthropological characteristics: brachycranial, hypsicranic, metriocranic, stenometopic, mestostaphyline, dolichuranic. The jaw is atrophied due to age. Kryptoprosopia, kryptozygia, plano-occipital because of the intentional formation. Small processus mastoideus, medium large tubera parietalia, 4 ossa suturarum on the left side, 3 on the right side of sutura lamboidea. Apertura piriformis is deep, the lower part is anthropine. Both sides of the alveolar ridge are closed, all the teeth have fallen out in lifetime. The palate is low.

<u>Grave No. 5</u>. The skull without the right parietal and the basal part, and the fragmentary skeletal bones of a 35 year old woman. Anthropological characteristics of the skull: dolichocranial, metriocranic,

eurymetopic, hypsiconchic, mesorrhine, brachyuranic, orthognathous, kryptoprosopic, kryptozygia, narrow sutura sphaenoparietalis, small tubera parietalia. The fossa canina is filled, the alveolar ridge is of parabolic, the palate is medium high. Two caries media on the teeth.

Grave No. 14. The complete skull of a 55 year old woman. The left temporal part is fractured. The skull was formed with double bandages. Anthropological characteristics: mesocranial, orthocranial, tapeinocranic, metriocranic, euryprosopic, mesorene, leptorene, mesoconchic, platyrrhine, brachystaphyline, dolichuranic, mesognathous. The form of the skull is rhomboidal-ovoidal. Kryptoprosopic, plano-occipital, narrow sutura sphaenoparietalis, medium large tubera parietalia, os incae monopartitum, very wide apertura piriformis, the lower part is anthropine, deep fossa canina, 7 cm long osteoma on the tabula externa of the left part of the forehead. 11 teeth have fallen out in lifetime, caries on the first praemolar on the left side. Mesodentes.

Grave No. 23. The calotte and two femura of a c. 40 year old woman. Anthropological characteristics of the skull: mesocranial, metrioeurymetopic, sphaenoidal, narrow forehead flattened by the intentional formation. Plano-occipital, large tubera parietalia, small tubera frontalia.

68. Nikitsch (Füles) (Burgenland, Deutschenkreus district). Graves of the Migration Period were found in 1925. Later J. Bayer and V. Lenzelter (1930) tried to locate the cemetery. V. Lebzelter excavated 23 graves that year, and later 29 more in collaboration with A. Ohrenberger. The skull found in grave No. 2a was intentionally formed. Archaeologists ascribed the cemetery to the Langobards, but anthropological examination indicates the Frankish-Thüringian ethnic group (I. Kiszely, 1976). The find was described by G. Müller in 1945 and 1936, who considered the skeleton to that of a man. The later examination proved it to be the skeleton of a 40 year old woman.

Anthropological characteristics of the skull: brachycranial, chamaecranial, tapeinocranic, stenometopic, eury-mesoprosopic, chamaeconchic, leptorrhine, dolichuranic, orthognathous. Form of the skull: sphaenoides. Phaenoprosopic, phaenozygia, plano-occipital, narrow sutura sphaenoparietalis, small glabella, rounded genial process, ossa suturarum on the right side of sutura lambdoidea, os incae bipartitum, small tubera frontalia due to the formation, rectangular orbits, the root of the nasal bone is slightly flattened, symmetrically narrow apertura piriformis, filled fossa canina, torus sagittalis on the palate, rounded foramen occipitale magnum. Two teeth have fallen out in lifetime, caries on three teeth.

69. Burgstall "Ruine Kromsegg" (Burgenland, Schiltern district). The grave of a 5-6 year old child was discovered by chance during E. Beninger's excavations at Loisbachtal in 1939. It is not known what archaeological finds came from the grave, only a note was to be found with the bones in the Naturhistorisches Museum: "Kinderskelett gefunden in inneren Vorwall bei der Wasserreibe".

The whole skeleton was recovered. The morphological characteristics indicate that it belonged to a girl. Anthropological characteristics of the skull: brachy-mesocranial, hypsicranial, macrocranial, medium narrow forehead, eurymetopic, orthognathous, hypereuryprosopic, hypereuryen, hyper-chamaerrhine, mesostaphyline, brachyuranic. The cranial bones are rather thick. Form of the skull: rhomboidal-birsoidal. Kryptoprosopic, kryptozygia, narrow forehead due to the intentional formation, medium large tubera frontalia, large tubera parietalia. Os epiptericum. Medium wide apertura piriformis, the lower part is vaulting, spina nasalis anterior is 2 (Brca's size), medium deep fossa canina, medium wide porus acusticus, its form is slanting oval. Rounded mentum, medium large foramen occipitale magnum, open sutura metopica, ossa Wormiana, 2 on the right side. Occlusion: labidont.

The skull suffered extreme formation carried out longitudinally with circular bandages. Basion-antibasion line: 146 mm, Oetteking-Ginzburg-Zhirov index: 104.11-hypermacrocranic. Oetteking angle: 72.5°.

The skull is likely to have belonged to a Goth.

INTENTIONALLY FORMED SKULLS FROM THE TERRITORY OF THE RUGII (LOWER AUSTRIA AND MORAVIA), AND THE VICINITY OF VIENNA

1. Atzgersdorf (at Liesing near Vienna). The second intentionally formed skull found in Austria, in 1846. Published by A. Retzius and L. Fitzinger in 1853.

2. Grafenwörth (Tulln district, Lower Austria). The site is on the southern part of Rugiland. The people buried here preceded the Langobards, and perhaps they were the Rugii themselves or the Heruli. The cemetery was discovered in 1921 and was excavated by E. Kloiber who discovered 18 graves. The first archaeological description was published by E. Beninger in 1948 (Fundberichte aus Osterreich III, p. 167). Later A. Lippert republished it (1968) using E. Kloibert's anthropological data. Two skulls found in the cemetery were intentionally formed.

3. Laa a.d. Thaya (Lower Austria). A badly preserved skull of a woman. It is in the Naturhistorisches Museum, but it is not restored yet and no anthropological examination can be carried out on it. Archaeological publication by E. Beninger, 1929.

4. Hobersdorf (Lower Austria, Mistelbach district). The skeleton of a man has been published by W. Ehgartner in Mitscha-Märheim's paper (1953). It was damaged and was lying 400 metres from the Wien-Poysdorf road. At first the skeleton was considered to be that of a Langobard, later it was ascribed to earlier peoples (H. Mitscha-Märheim, 1969). The skull is fragmentary, and is medium formed. The archaeologist mentioned another intentionally formed skull unearthed later in a grave on the same area, but it has not been sent to the museum or been examined by experts.

5. Deutsch-Altenburg (Carnuntum). A stray find of unknown date in Dr Toldt's possession. Published by A. Schliz, 1905.

6. Feuersbrunn b. Grafenegg (Lower Austria). The intentionally formed skull was ploughed up in 1820. J. Fitzinger published it in detail in 1853. The skull has been lost but J. Fitzinger's authentic sketches are of great value (A. Schliz, 1905).

7. Wien-Salvatorgasse. A. Neumann, archaeologist of the Stadtmuseum Wien, directed excavations in 1951 of the Roman remains, and found three skeletons with extremely formed skulls. They were published by H. M. Pacher in 1965. The skulls, contrary to the published analysis, belonged to women, and can be ascribed to the Goths, not to the Langobards (I. Kiszely, 1976).

8. Wien-Mariahilferstrasse (alternative name Mariahilfergürtel). 20 graves ascribed to the Langobards were discovered at the end of the last century. Anthropological examination indicated that they were Gothic. One of the skulls was intentionally formed, and is now on exhibition in the Stadtmuseum Wien. Published by J. Fitzinger, 1853; M. Much, 1898; A. Schliz, 1905 and E. Beninger, 1938.

9. Wien-Simmering. An extremely formed skull was found in a cemetery ascribed to the Goths and the Alans. A drawing and a description were published by H. Mitscha-Märheim, 1963. The skull was lost during the Second World War, and only the data and photographs have survived.

10. Wien-Baden. An intentionally formed skull was found in a cave on Calvary Hill between 1823 and 1829. The finds were described by G. Rasoumovsky. J. Fitzinger could not find it in 1853.

11. Wien-Mödling. Intentionally formed skulls of a woman and a child were discovered in recent years according to oral information from H. Mitscha-Märheim. The finds have not been sent to the Naturhistorisches Museum, and their whereabouts are unknown.

12. Novy Saldorf (Znoimo district, Moravia). 75 graves were excavated in 1923-1924. They were dated to the 6th century by E. Beninger in 1933, and to the end of the 5th century A.D. by J. Cervinka in 1936-1937. The finds including the 7 intentionally formed skulls were published by A. Lorenzova in 1963. The bones are in Clovek Museum in Prague. The intentionally formed skulls were found in the following graves: 8, X_1, X_2, X_3, X_4, 30, X_5.

13. Velatice, Zadni Pulany ul. (Moravia, Brno district). The excavations began in 1936 (I. Cervinka, 1939, J. Paulik, 1950). 20 graves have been found, 3 of which contained intentionally formed skulls. Published by J. Jelinek, 1960. Later A. Lorenzova re-published it together with three new skulls (1960-1962). Three intentionally formed skulls belonged to women, two to men, and one to a child.

14. Brnenské Ivanovice (Brno district). The finds came from P. Richter. They were first mentioned by J. Cervinka (1936, 1939) and E. Beninger and H. Freising (1933). The calotte of the adult woman was examined by A. Lorencova in 1963.

15. Znoimo. The excavation of a large cemetery was begun in 1870 (M. Trapp, 1872; J. Cervinka, 1902; J. Palliardi, 1888; E. Beninger and H. Freising, 1939). Only one intentionally formed skull of an adult man has survived. It was deposited in Clovek Museum in Prague, and later published by A. Lorenzova in 1963.

16. Vícemilice (Bucovice district). Workers in the clay-pit found 4 graves from the Early Migration Period in 1912, and one of them they preserved. (M. Chleborad, 1941; A. Rzehák, 1918; E. Beninger and H. Freising, 1933.) The intentionally formed skull of a 20 year old woman was examined by A. Lorenzova in 1959 and in 1963. The find is in Moravské Museum in Brno.

17. Raksice (Krumlov district). An isolated grave of a woman was found in 1924 (E. Beninger and H. Freising, 1933; J. Cervinka, 1939). The intentionally formed skull was published by J. Jelinek in 1960, A. Lorenzova in 1963 and I. Kiszely in 1976.

18. Sedlesovice (Znoimo district). The medium formed skull of a mature man was found in 1963 and was sent to the Anthrop. Ustav in Brno. It was published by A. Lorenzova in 1963 and by I. Kiszely in 1976.

19. Polkovice (Kojetin district). An isolated grave was found in 1929 (J. Cervinka, 1933; J. Skutil, 1931; E. Beninger and H. Freising, 1933). The considerably formed skull of a 20-30 year old woman is now in Clovek Museum in Prague. Published by A. Lorenzova, 1958, 1963.

20. Vacenovice (Kyjova district). An isolated grave was found in 1954 (A. Lorenzova, M. Pospisil and L. Kalus, 1957). The medium formed skull of a young adult woman was first examined by L. Kalus and then by A. Lorenzova in 1963. The find is in the county museum of Gottwaldov.

21. Vyskov (Brno district). 50 graves have been excavated from the Eneolithic, Bronze Age and the Migration Periods. The excavations were carried out in 1938 under G. Krivanek's direction. 18 graves date from the Migration Period (J. Skutil, 1946). The skull found in the 18th and 42nd graves, both belonging to women, were intentionally formed. Published by M. Stloukal in 1965.

22. Nova Ves (Pohorelic district). The intentionally formed skull (calva only) of an 11-13 year old girl was found in 1956. The anthropological examination of the find was carried out by J. Jelinek in 1958 and A. Lorenzova in 1963. The find is now in the Moravske Museum in Brno.

23. Slapanice (Brno district). An isolated grave from the Early Migration Period was found in 1934 (J. Poulik, 1937, 1941; J. Cervinka, 1936). The calva of a child (infant II) was examined by A. Lorenzova in 1963.

24. Staré Mesto (Uherské-Hradiste district). In grave no. 43 of a great cemetery from the Migration Period containing 89 graves, the skeleton of a 30-40 year old woman was unearthed in 1948. The skull was intentionally formed. The cemetery belonged, probably, to the Heruli or the Merovingians (J. Pavelcik, 1949). Anthropological publica-

tion was by A. Lorenzova in 1963, 1964. The skeleton of the adult woman was also mentioned later by J. Cervinka (1939).

26. Drslavice (Uherski Brod district). An isolated skeleton of a woman with a formed skull was found in 1933 (J. Cervinka, 1936). It was anthropologically examined by A. Lorenzova in 1963.

27. Saratice (Slavkov district). The site has been known since 1928. Two graves were published in 1928, eight in 1948-1949 by J. Poulik, and 26 Langobard graves were mentioned by C. Stana in 1954. A total of 36 graves was excavated (J. Cervinka, 1936, 1937). The skeleton lying in grave No. 21b had intentionally formed skull. It was published by A. Lorenzova in 1963.

THE FINAL AREAS OF EXPANSION OF THE CUSTOM

BOHEMIA

1. Praha-Podbaba (Bohemia). For the first few years the finds made at the Podbaba brick factory were destroyed, until at last in 1891 five graves were discovered and the material was sent to J. Pic, who examined and published them (1891-1892). Later excavations yielded 41 more graves. L. Niederle published 8 skeletons in 1891 under the title: "Die neuentdeckte Gräber von Podbaba und der erste Künstliche deformierte prähistorische Schädel aus Böhmen". According to him the graves belonged to "the Marcomannic population resident there". The skull of the 7th grave was intentionally formed, and belonged to an 18 year old woman.

2. Zaluzi (Praha-vychod) (from 1940: Celakovice). L. Hajek discovered 5 graves in 1930-1931, and later J. Schranil uncovered 52 graves (1932). The archaeological analysis of the cemetery was made by L. Franz in 1935, while the intentionally formed skulls found in graves 28 and 46 (women) were published by J. Maly in 1935. All the human bones except the two intentionally formed skulls were destroyed during the Second World War.

3. Klucov (Cesky Brod district, east of Prague). Several graves from the Migration Period were found in 1951. J. Kabát rescued 5 graves in 1952 and later the number of graves reached 23. (S. Svoboda, 1965; J. Kudrnac, 1952, 1953.) One of the first five graves contained an intentionally formed skull, and was labelled grave no. 1 later. The find was published by E. Vlcek in 1952. The head of the young woman was medium formed.

4. Luzec nad Vltavou (Melnik district). The Archaeological Institute in Prague financed excavations in 1955 on the site. O. Kytliková uncovered several graves dating from the 5th-6th centuries B.C. according to the archaeologists. In grave no. 18, a double grave, the skull of a child was intentionally formed. It was published by J. Chochol in 1969.

5. Budyna-Budin (on the River Eger, Raudnitz district). An intentionally formed skull was published by H. Matiekga in 1894. The skull has been lost (Rozpravy Ceské Akad. Cis. Frant. Jos. Praha. XI, p. 26).

CENTRAL GERMANY, THURINGIA

6. Grossörner-Molmeck (Kreis Hettstedt). An intentionally formed skull was found in 1936. It has never been published, only some photographs have been taken of it. The find was lost during the Second World War (L. Scholl, 1961).

7. Hedersleben (Kr. Quedlinburg). The intentionally formed skull of an 18-20 year old woman is now in the Quedlinburg Museum. Archaeological publication by K. Zeigel, 1939; anthropological analysis by L. Schott, 1961.

8. Lützen (Kr. Weissenfels, formerly Merseburg). The intentionally formed skull of a 35-40 year old woman was found in grave no. 2. Archaeological publication was made by K. Zeigel, 1939, and N. Niklosson, 1929; anthropological examination was carried out by L. Schott, 1961.

9. Obermöllern (Kr. Naumburg). The intentionally formed skull of an old woman. The cemetery was excavated by F. Holter in 1925. In his publication he presents the description and photograph of the skull found in grave V. Later the find was published by L. Schott (1961). The skull from grave VI was badly preserved (probably an old woman). F. Holter published its photograph, but the skull has not been restored and described. The detailed publication was also made by L. Schott (1961).

10. Rathewitz (Kr. Naumburg). The intentionally formed skull of a middle-aged woman was published by R. Schmidt in 1955 and 1956; the full anthropological analysis was carried out by L. Schott in 1961.

11. Stössen (now Kreis Wiessenfels, formerly Kreis Hochenmölsen). The skeleton of a 35-40 year old woman, lying in the grave no. 36 of a Thüringian cemetery had an intentionally formed skull (K. Ziegel, 1939). The anthropological analysis was carried out by L. Schott in 1961.

12. Dossenheim (near Heidelberg). Published by B. Heukemes, H. Hoepke and W. Kindler, 1956. The anthropological analysis was carried out by H. Hoepke in 1959.

13. Naumburg-Schönburgerstrasse. The skull found in grave IV of the great Nagel Naumburg cemetery ascribed to the Thüringians was intentionally formed. The find was destroyed in the Second World War, and no anthropological examination was carried out on it. Mentioned by G. Mildenberger and J. Werner, 1956.

14. Ingersleben (Kr. Erfurt), The skull found in grave no. 2 of the cemetery, probably belonging to a woman, was intentionally formed. The archaeological finds were published by H. Kaufmann in 1953-1954 and D. Drost in 1955. No detailed anthropological description has been published. The skull is in the Gotha Museum.

15. Grossfahner (Kr. Erfurt). An intentionally formed skull of a woman was found in a cemetery dating from the 6th century A.D. Published by G. Florschütz, 1934 and K. Gerhardt, 1939. The find was lost in the Second World War.

16. Weimar-Cranachstrasse (Kr. Zauch-Belzig). Two intentionally formed skulls of women were found. Published by R. Hoffman, 1939. Both finds were lost during the Second World War.

17. Phöben (Kr. Zauch-Belzig, Brandenburg). The intentionally formed skull of an old woman was published by R. Hoffmann in 1939. The find was destroyed in the Potzdam Museum during the Second World War.

18. Schöningen-Salzstrasse (Braumschweig). The intentionally formed skull of a woman was published by G. Theringer in 1939. Later J. Nemeskéry republished it in Mitt. d. Naturhistorische Museum (1977).

19. Sittichenbach (Kr. Querfurt). The intentionally formed skull of a woman was found in 1958 or 1959. It has not yet been properly examined. The photograph and the most important data on the skull have been published by L. Schott in 1961.

SOUTH GERMANY: Rhine Valley

20. Köln (St. Ursula Church). The calvarium of a woman's skull has survived. Published by H. Schaffhausen in 1866, 1876, 1879.

21. Meckenheim (Kr. Bonn). The intentionally formed skull of a woman was published by H. Schaffhausen (1879), A. Schliz (1905) and K. Gerhardt (1965).

22. Niederholm (South of Mainz, in Rheinhessen). The skull of an old woman was found in 1862. The anthropological characteristics were published by A. Schliz (1905) and A. Ecker (1866). The skull has since been lost.

23. Darmstadt. H. Schaffhausen mentioned and described the find in 1879 but A. Schliz does not even mention it in 1905 (K. Gerhardt, 1965).

24. Heilbronn (on the River Neckar). The intentionally formed skull of an adult woman was found in an Alamannic cemetery excavated in Rosenberg strasse (Clussische Brauerei). Anthropological analysis was carried out by A. Schliz, 1905.

25. Strassburg. Three intentionally formed skulls have been found. They were labelled "Weisstortum".

    i. Calvarium from grave no. 65 in a Roman cemetery. According to H. Ullrich (1957) it belonged to a 45-50 year old woman. It was published by W. Waldeyer in 1881 in A. Staub's paper.

    ii. An intentionally formed skull was found in another grave in the same cemetery.

    iii. An intentionally formed skull, labelled "Strassenbahndepot Kronenburg" was found in 1931. It seems to have been an isolated grave of an adult woman belonging to the Frankish ethnic group. The anthropological analysis of the find was carried out by H. Ullrich in 1957.

26. Dachstein (Dep. Strassburg). A Merovingian cemetery was found in 1955. The first grave contained the intentionally formed skull of a woman. Published by H. Ullrich in 1957 (K. Gerhardt, 1965).

27. Straubing (Niederbayern). A grave with Merovingian archaeological finds has been excavated. The badly preserved skull of a woman was intentionally formed. Published by J. Keim in 1928 and by K. Gerhardt in 1965.

28. Irlmauth (Gemeinde Barbing, east of Regensburg). The grave no. 33 in the Kiesgrube-Hölzl cemetery, ascribed to the Merovingians, contained the skeletal bones and the intentionally formed skull of a man. The finds were published by K. Gerhardt in 1965. The skeleton found in 1939 is now in the Regensburg Museum with the inventory number 1939/441 253.

29. Eltheim-Gemeindekiesgrube (east of Regensburg). The inventory number of the skull is Sk 172. There were no associated grave goods. The finds were discovered earlier than the Irlmauth one. The frontal and the facial parts are whole but the calvaria is represented only by a part of the parietal. Intentional formation is of great extent. It seems to have belonged to a man. The find was published by K. Gerhardt in 1965. As for the proper ethnical grouping, G. Kurth wrote: "dass der Eltheimer ein iranische Alane sein könnte"..."Dieses Volk brachte die Deformation schon aus seinen Wolgareiche mit und fach sicher mehrfach die Gelegenheit, in botmassigen Kriegerhaufen oder Söldnerscharen den Donauweg zu benutzen...." (p. 23).

30. Altenerding (München). A great cemetery was uncovered in the late 1960s. Three skulls (graves 513, 125 and one uncertain) were intentionally formed. The one in grave 513 was formed to a great extent, the other two (also women) had suffered medium formation. Published by H. Helmuth in 1973.

BURGUNDY (Switzerland and France)

31. Bel-Air-Chesaux (Lausanne). The find was discovered by Trojon at the beginning of the last century. The first description of the intentionally formed skull of the c. 40 year old man was written by W. His and L. Rütimeyer in 1864, though they did not notice the intentional head formation. In the same time they considered the skull in grave 68 to be formed, but this skull has subsequently been lost. The publication of the finds was later made by M. Sauter, 1939.

32. Genthod (Geneva). A badly preserved skull was found without grave-goods on the banks of Lake Leman in 1927. It must have belonged to a 50 year old man. Published by M. Sauter, 1939.

33. Gaillard (Geneva). An intentionally formed skull was found by E. Pittard in a Burgundian grave. The skull, that of a mature man, was published by M. Sauter in 1939.

34. Villy (at Reignier, Haute-Savoie). The finds were published by L. Gosse in 1955, A. Schliz and M. Sauter (1939) and also by E. Salin in 1952.

35. Annecy (Haute-Savoye). The find was described by Marteaux and Le Roux in 1902, and later by M. Sauter in 1939.

36. Voiteur (in Jura, 10 km north-west of Lons-le-Saunnier). The intentionally formed skull was first described by P. Broca in 1864 (Bull. Soc. d'Anthropologie de Paris, V, p. 385) and E. Chantre (1880). Later it was published by A. Schliz (1905) and M. Sauter (1939).

37. Corveissiat (c. Ain, 17 km south-east of Treffort). Two intentionally formed skulls were found in Burgundian graves. They were described by E. Chantre in 1881 (Révue d'Anthropologie II, Ser. 4) and M. Sauter (1939).

38. Mesocco-Benabbia (Graubünden Kanton). The find was made by R. Boldini in 1843 among graves from the Migration Period. The intentionally formed skull of a mature man, found in grave 2, was published by O. Schlaginhaufen in 1944.

OTHER AREAS OF EUROPE

39. Marseille-Rue de la République. Two intentionally formed skulls were found, dating from post-Roman times. They were mentioned by J. Fallot in 1881 (Bull. Soc. d'Anthropologie de Paris III, Ser. 4, pp. 807-811) and E. Chantre in 1886.

40. Złota (Poland). B. Miszkiewicz published a skull in 1885. Its proper ethnical grouping cannot be determined.

41. The latest and most northerly intentionally formed skulls in Europe were found in Sweden. The finds were published by I. Kiszely and I. Hankó in 1974. Skull No. 1 is labelled St Ihre, Hellvi parish, and was found in Gotland; skull No. 2 with the label Kvie, Eksta parish was also found in Gotland; skull No. 3 with the label Havor, Hablingbo parish was found in Gotland as well. The finds date from the "Viking Age" i.e. 800-1050 A.D. All the three skulls belonged to women who were perhaps three of those Heruli, mentioned by Procopius of Caesarea in his History of the Wars (VI.15), who returned to Scandinavia.

Scholars have in the past been unable to arrive at an agreed standpoint concerning the problem of Central and Western European intentional head formation. The difficulty lay in the apparently mongoloid characteristics which were ascribed to the Huns, a population practically unknown to the European scientists. J. Werner mentions it again and again (p. 14):

> "...dabei mit einer mongolischen Komponente und mit echtem hunnischen Einschlag rechnen kann...die Hunnen in diesen Gebiete ihre Spuren hinterlassen haben".

It was supposed that all the European intentionally formed skulls belonged to the descendants of the people married into Hun families.

> "In Lichte dieser Funde gewinnt ein von den Anthropologen des 19. Jh. immer wieder angeführter Passus bei Sidonius Apollinaris an Gewicht, der gern für das Vorhandensein von Schädeldeformation bei den europäischen Hunnen herangezogen wurde. Der Senator aus der Auvergne schreibt in seiner Schilderung der Hunnen vom

> Jahre 466: 'consurgit in arctum massa rotunda caput, geminis sub fronte cavernus visus adest oculis absentibus'...." (p. 16).

According to the earlier defective theories (p. 17):

> "the Thuringians from Central Germany, the Langobards from Moravia, the 'Pre-Bavarians' from Bohemia, and the Gepidae and the Ostrogoths from the Crimea all lived in Attila's Empire and the custom of head formation was taken over from the ruling nomadic groups" (J. Werner, 1956).

He explained the fact that the custom is not practised by the Alamanni and the Franks by suggesting that they had had no direct contact with the Huns. The decline of the custom is connected with that of the Hun Empire, its dissemination with the greatest area conquered by the Huns. Werner finishes his essay by saying (p. 18):

> "In einer andergearteten Umwelt wurde dieses im wahrsten Sinne des Wortes exotische Kulturelement in dem Augenblick wieder abgestossen als das hunnische Grossreich nach dem Tode Attilas zusammenstürtzte".

Any science which lacks a basis of plentiful and unambiguous data tends to lead its exponents into drawing broad and seemingly solid general conclusions; this is the Hegelian stage of thesis. As more data accumulates and original theories lose their validity and even "certain" data becomes ambiguous—the stage of antithesis. All these doubts yield in turn the synthesis, providing solid and reliable facts, sifted through criticism and supported by the evidence of the finds.

The recent period, including J. Werner (1956), has been that of thesis. The finds are now accumulating from day to day: we cannot keep pace with all the recent finds all over the world. About 1,000 intentionally formed skulls from 260 sites are listed in this paper but the total number of finds dating from historical times is much greater and is still growing in Eurasia.

This accumulation has not only caused quantitative changes, but has also broadened the time scale and the geographical extension of the custom. The first intentionally formed skulls discovered in the Near East date from the 6th millennium B.C., or perhaps even earlier in the 8th millennium, and are connected with similar customs in Africa (Ethiopia).

The burials which have been best preserved from prehistoric times are those from towns, so their discovery is largely accidental and does not reflect the real territorial extension of the custom. The only reliable and positive data is that the custom does not go further than the Iranian Highlands, is unknown in Siberia and also, in the earlier periods, on the northern coast of the Black Sea.

The traces of an early infiltration into Europe between 2,300-2,200 and 1,900 B.C. are becoming more and more distinct. The custom may have been carried by merchants but it is also possible that it was carried by the same people who brought the Indo-European language into Europe. The finds are too few to prove this theory, but the expansion of the custom coincides with the territory inhabited by the first peoples who spoke the Indo-European language in Europe. This theory can be included among the unnumerable hypotheses trying, so far in vain, to give a true picture of the Indo-European peoples.

The custom of intentional head formation soon arrived in the Caucasus (Bronze Age, Ordzhokinidze), where it survived for a long time up to the present day, and spread to the surrounding areas. I myself have seen people with intentionally formed heads at Jezids near Djebel Sinjar in Iraq and in the surrounding villages such as Bahsany and Bashiqa. The forming cradle is called by the Armenians "mehed", and by the Assurians "darjushta", and it is also used by other peoples, e.g. the Osets.

The Goths, Alans and Sarmatians peopling the northern coast of the Black Sea took over the custom soon afterwards. The Huns on their way from the west coast of Lake Baikal towards Europe met head-forming peoples of Iranian racial type (the Kenkol group). The Huns absorbed them and went on towards Europe, carrying them along. The invasion of the Huns drove the peoples living on the northern shores of the Black Sea (the Goths, Alans and Gepids) into Central Europe, and thus formed the first centre in Central Europe, in the Carpathian Basin. Here both men and women practised the custom, sometimes drawing their heads out to extreme lengths.

The second European centre was in the territory of the Rugii, where they and the Heruli, two archaeologically ill-defined peoples, practised the custom. Their territory coincided with the area in which the custom of head formation was practised. The Langobards did not form their heads, as has long been supposed; all such finds belonged in fact to the Rugii (Steinbrunn, Nikitsch, Wien, etc.).

Some finds are also encountered north-west of the territory of the Rugii, among the Thüringians, Merovingians and sometimes among the Burgundians and rarely also the Alamanni and Franks. The northernmost skulls were unearthed in Gotland, belonging, perhaps, to Heruli who had returned to their native land from the territory of the Rugii.

The custom survived in some areas in a modified form, e.g. in the Dinarian Alps among the Albanians, in the Caucasus, in the South of France, in North Mesopotamia and so on. No connections can be found, and perhaps none should be sought, between them. Head formation was a fashion, intended to make people more elegant and nobler, as we can see on their descendents living today.

We do not discuss in this work the morphological changes caused by extreme "deformation" of the skull, or the mental injuries. The topics discussed in detail by E. Dingwall (1931) and H. Helmuth (1970). However it is anthropologically noticeable that intentional head formation caused compensational growth, leading to pseudo-mongoloid characteristics in the skull: the zygomatic processes were made more outstanding, the root of the mose was flattened, the face too was flatter and so on. These changes have misled experts into false theories about the Huns, calling them mongoloid or at least "Tartarians".

The custom is purely a question of fashion, the historical-anthropological importance of which is that it can be ascribed to ethnic groups and so can help in the detection of contacts between peoples. It can also serve as a proof of the unity and undivisibility of mankind and of the fact that similar thoughts (and also fashions) can develop independently of territory, race and nationality or ethnic group. The constantly growing quantity of information provided by new finds emphasises our error when we try to give firm and far-reaching solutions to problems when our information is in fact too limited for the purpose.

Our aim has been and will be in the near future to publish reliable and true facts in this field, so that they may serve as elements for those who will make future syntheses.

Table 1 Artificially deformed skulls from Eridu (Tell Abu Shahrain)

Measurement numbers after Martin	Characteristics	Skull Number							
		1	2	3	4	5	6	7	8
1	Glabello-occipital length (g–op)	180	179	191	184	175	191	180	199
3	Glabello-lambda length (g–l)	180	177	189	183	174	191	180	194
8	Max. breadth of cranium (eu–eu)	128	135	135	123	133	142	138	143
9	Anterior forehead breadth (ft–ft)	98	95	90	97	99	101	99	101
10	Posterior forehead breadth (co–co)	113	118	110	123	123	121	118	120
11	Biauricular breadth (au–au)	105	110	110	120	108	107	116	133
13	Mastoideal breadth (ms–ms)	100?	94	99	102	–	89	97	135
17	Basis-bregmatic height (ba–b)	130?	106	117	–	–	101	112	–
20	Auricular-bregma height (po–b)	100?	90?	87?	98	99	76	94?	121?
23	Horizontal circumference	509?	523	508	535	525	558	530	557
24	Transverse arc (po–po)	271	276	276	306	265	285	285	310
25	Sagittal skull arch (n–o)	367	362	358	370?	–	390	351	–
32/1	Nasion-bregma angle	45°	61°	48°	52°	55°	–	–	–
32/a	Tangential angle	67°	63°	64°	47°	57°	–	–	–
40	Nasion-prothion length (ba–pr)	–	166	145	–	–	99?	–	–
42	Lower-face length (ba–gn)	–	105	121	–	–	132?	–	–
43	Upper-face breadth (fmt–fmt)	105	107	107	110	110	108	–	107
45	Bizygomatic breadth (zy–zy)	130?	118	122	134	127	126	101	143
46	Middle-face breadth (zm–zm)	102	92	99	97	95	–	–	76?
47	Nasion-granthion height (n–gn)	112	93	120	111?	111	101	–	–
48	Nasion-prosthion height (n–pr)	66	55	72	67	63	51	–	–
51	Orbital breadth (mf–sk)	39 39	39 38	41–40	– 40	37 40	40 39	–	41 –

(continued)

Table 1 (contd.)

Measurement numbers after Martin	Characteristics	Skull Number							
		1	2	3	4	5	6	7	8
52	Orbital height (or–m)	27 29	19? 23?	33–31	34	30 29	37 40	–	34 –
54	Nasal breadth	23	23	23	25	25?	21	–	–
55	Nasal height (n–ns)	48	40	56	51	43	–	–	–
65	Condylar breadth (kdl-kdl)	107	107	107	132?	111	–	118	–
68	Mandibular length	113	90	109	111	–	102	99	100
69	Mentum height (id-gn)	29	27	37	30	35?	35	26	30
72	Total face angle	82°	72°	84°	92°?	79°	–	–	–
73	Medium facial angle	84°	72°	83°	91°?	79°	–	–	–
79	Angulus mandubulae	122°	118°	116°	117°	111°	117°	115°	–
47:45	Morphological face index	86.50	78.81	98.36	82.84	87.40	80.16	–	–
48:45	Upper-face index	50.77?	46.61	59.02	50.00	49.61	40.48	–	–
52:51	Orbital index	69.23– 74.36	48.71– 60.52	80.49– 80.00	–85.00 –	81.08– 72.50	32.50– 102.50	–	82.92–
54:55	Nasal index	47.91	57.50	41.07	49.01	58.14	–	–	–
8:1	Cranial index (Garson)	71.11	75.42	70.68	66.85	75.00	74.34	76.67	71.85
20:1	Length-height index	55.55	50.28	45.55?	53.26	56.57	39.80	52.22	60.80
20:8	Breadth-height index	78.12	66.67	64.44	79.67	74.44	53.52	68.12	84.62
9:8	Transversal index	76.56	70.37	66.67	78.85	74.44	71.12	71.74	70.63

Table 2. Measurements of artificially deformed skulls from Szentes-Bökény, Hungary

No.*	Characteristics	Szentes-Bökény Grave No.		
		11	15	17
1	Glabello-occipital length (g-op)	180	182	183
3	Glabello-lambda length (g-l)	-	180	177
8	Max. breadth of cranium (eu-eu)	152	136	143
9	Anterior forehead breadth (ft-ft)	-	-	96
10	Posterior forehead breadth (co-co)	130	122	117
11	Biauricular breadth (au-au)	128	120	123
13	Mastoidal breadth (ms-ms)	113	108	110
17	Basis-bregmatic height (ba-b)	-	-	-
20	Auricular-bregma height (po-b)	124	-	122
23	Horizontal circumference	-	-	525
24	Transverse arc (po-po)	-	-	310
25	Sagittal skull arch (n-o)	-	-	380?
32/1	Nasion-bregma angle	-	-	64°
32/a	Tangential angle	-	-	76°
40	Basion-prothion length (ba-pr)	-	-	-
42	Lower-face length (ba-gn)	-	-	-
43	Upper-face breadth (fmt-fmt)	-	-	104
45	Bizygomatic breadth (zy-zy)	-	-	130
46	Middle-face breadth (zm-zm)	-	-	95
47	Nasion-gnathion height (n-gn)	-	-	113
48	Nasion-prosthion height (n-pr)	-	-	72
51	Orbital breadth (mf-ek)	-	-	38 35
52	Orbital height (or-m)	-	-	30 31
54	Nasal breadth	-	-	-
55	Nasal height (n-ns)	-	-	52
65	Condylar breadth (kdl-kdl)	130	120	122
68	Mandibular length	120	100	110
69	Mentum height (id-gn)	28	18	34
72	Total face angle	-	-	86°
73	Medium facial angle	-	-	84°
69	Angulus mandubulae	124°	115°	124°
47:45	Morphological face index	-	-	86.92
48:45	Upper face index	-	-	55.38
52:51	Orbital index	-	-	78.95 88.57
54:55	Nasal index	-	-	-
8:1	Cranial index (Garson)	84.44	74.72	78.57
20:1	Length-height index	68.89	-	67.03
20:8	Breadth-height index	81.58	-	85.31
9:9	Transversal index	-	-	67.13

Table 3. Measurements of artificially deformed skulls from the Roman Cemetery at Intercisa (Dunaujváros), Hungary

Measurement numbers after Martin	Characteristics	Intercisa Grave Numbers				
		210	600	1481	1485	1492
1	Glabello-occipital length (g-op)	162	185	158	165	179
3	Glabello-lambda length (g-l)	158	175	158	162	169
8	Max. breadth of cranium (eu-eu)	138	154	154	132	138
9	Anterior forehead breadth (ft-ft)	92	104	98	84	102
10	Posterior forehead breadth (co-co)	116	134	122	110	120
11	Biauricular breadth (au-au)	–	125	146	121	122
13	Mastoideal breadth (ms-ms)	–	107	132	111	110
17	Basis-bregmatic height (ba-b)	136	140	146	–	–
20	Auricular-bregma height (po-b)	112	126	107	110	106
23	Horizontal circumference	490	535	515	530	515
24	Transverse arc (po-po)	300?	367	310	330	316
25	Sagittal skull arch (n-o)	350	387	375	382	–
32/1	Nasion-bregma angle	54°	54°	54°	56°	–
32/a	Tangential angle	78°	82°	78°	66°	–
40	Basion-prostion length (ba-pr)	82	98	–	–	–
42	Lower-face length (ba-gn)	–	121	–	–	–
43	Upper-face breadth (fmt-fmt)	100	110	112	99	–
45	Bizygomatic breadth (zy-zy)	–	142	–	128?	–
46	Middle face breadth (zm-zm)	–	98	–	100?	–
47	Nasion-gnathion height (n-gn)	–	122	–	107	–
48	Nasion prosthion height (n-pr)	64	70	75	65	–
51	Orbital breadth (mf-ek)	–	42	37	37	–
52	Orbital height (or-m)	31	32	28	30	–

(Table continued)

Table 3 (contd.)

Measurement numbers after Martin	Characteristics	Intercisa Grave Numbers				
		210	600	1481	1485	1492
54	Nasal breadth	23	24	20	12	–
55	Nasal height (n–ns)	48	55	41	48	–
65	Condylar breadth (kdl–kdl)	–	132	–	103	–
68	Mandibular length	–	117	–	122	–
69	Mentum height (id–gn)	–	34	–	27	–
72	Total face angle	–	84°	75°	85°	–
73	Medium facial angle	–	86°	74°	88°	–
69	Angulus mandibulae	–	129°	–	123°	–
8:1	Cranial index (Garson)	85.18	83.24	97.46	80.00	77.09
20:1	Length-height index	69.14	68.10	67.72	66.67	59.21
20:8	Breadth-height index	81.16	81.81	69.48	83.33	76.81
9:8	Transversal index	66.67	67.53	63.64	63.64	73.91
47:45	Morphological face index	–	85.91	–	83.59 ?	–
48:45	Upper-face index	–	49.30	–	50.67	–
52:51	Orbital index	–	76.19 80.00	– 75.68	– 81.08	–
54:55	Nasal index	47.92	43.64	48.78	25.00	–

Table 4. Measurements of artificially deformed skulls from the Cemeteries at Burgstall (Austria), Rácalmás and Fertőszentmiklós (Hungary)

Measurement numbers after Martin	Characteristics	Burgstall (Burgenland)	Rácalmás Grave 133	Fertőszentmiklós
1	Glabello-occipital length (g-op)	163	157	173
3	Glabello-lambda length (g-l)	160	155	171
8	Max. breadth of cranium (eu-eu)	131	128	134
9	Anterior forehead breadth (ft-ft)	93	89	88
10	Posterior forehead breadth (co-co)	113	103	122
11	Biauricular breadth (au-au)	103	101	108
13	Mastoideal breadth (ms-ms)	93	108	96
17	Basis-bregmatic height (ba-b)	136	131	130
20	Auricular-bregma height (po-b)	124	110	111
23	Horizontal circumference	475	460	490
24	Transverse arc (po-po)	323	290	305
25	Sagittal skull arch (n-o)	375	322	365
32/1	Nasion-bregma angle	58°	61°	47°
32/a	Tangential angle	58°	58°	72°
40	Basion-prosthion length (ba-pr)	77	96	84
42	Lower-face length (ba-gn)	85	–	–
43	Upper-face breadth (fmt-fmt)	91	98	98
45	Bizygomatic breadth (zy-zy)	104	124 ?	125
46	Middle-face breadth (zm-zm)	72	94	86
47	Nasion-gnathion height (n-gn)	77	–	–
48	Nasion-prosthion height (n-pr)	43	67	68
51	Orbital breadth (mf-ek)	32 33	31 34	37 35
52	Orbital height (or-m)	36 37	27 28	30 28

(Table continued)

Table 4 (contd.)

Measurement numbers after Martin	Characteristics	Burgstall (Burgenland)		Rácalmás Grave 133		Fertőszentmikós	
54	Nasal breadth	20		20		24	
55	Nasal height (n-ns)	33		–		52	
65	Condylar breadth (kdl-kdl)	96		–		–	
68	Mandibular length	72		–		–	
69	Mentum height (id-gn)	23		–		–	
72	Total face angle	85°		88°		82°	
73	Medium facial angle	83°		87°		82°	
69	Angulus mandubulae	128°		–		–	
47:45	Morphological face index	74.04		–		–	
48:45	Upper-face index	41.35		54.03 ?		54.40	
52:51	Orbital index	112.50	112.12	87.10	82.35	81.08	80.00
54:55	Nasal index	60.61		–		46.15	
8:1	Cranial index (Garson)	80.37		81.53		77.46	
20:1	Length-height index	76.07		70.06		63.58	
20:8	Breadth-height index	94.66		85.94		82.84	
9:8	Transversal index	82.30		69.53		65.67	

Table 5. Measurements of artificially deformed skulls from Nikitsch and Steinbrunn

Measurement numbers after Martin		Nikitsch		Steinbrunn	
		Grave 2/a	Grave 3/a	Grave 16	Grave 17
1	Glabello-occipital length (g–op)	177	182	173 ?	172
3	Glabello-lambda length (g–l)	173	174	–	169
8	Max. breadth of cranium (eu–eu)	142	140	133	143
9	Anterior forehead breadth (ft–ft)	93	94	–	92
10	Posterior forehead breadth (co–co)	119	115	115 ?	121
11	Biauricular breadth (au–au)	123	120	121	122
13	Mastoideal breadth (ms–ms)	98	103	107	107
17	Basis-bregmatic height (ba–b)	114	–	–	129
20	Auricular-bregma height (po–b)	100	119	117	115
23	Horizontal circumference	520	518	–	503
24	Transverse arc (po–po)	302	300	312	308
25	Sagittal skull arch (n–o)	363	365	–	353
32/1	Nasion-bregma angle	47°	48°	–	–
32/a	Tangential angle	77°	78°	–	–
40	Basion-prothion length (ba–pr)	94	–	–	89 ?
42	Lower-face length (ba–gn)	115	–	–	103
43	Upper-face breadth (fmt–fmt)	110	105	–	–
45	Bizygomatic breadth (zy–zy)	128	122	–	–
46	Middle-face breadth (zm–zm)	88	91	–	–
47	Nasion-granthion height (n–gn)	109	–	–	102 ?
48	Nasion-prosthion height (n–pr)	66	68	–	60
51	Orbital breadth (mf–ek)	34 42	37 40	–	–
52	Orbital height (or–m)	30 32	30 30	–	–
54	Nasal breadth	20	26	–	25

(Table continued)

Table 5 (contd.)

Measurement numbers after Martin	Characteristics	Nikitsch	Steinbrunn		
		Grave 2/a	Grave 3/1	Grave 16	Grave 17
55	Nasal height (n-ns)	50	50	–	–
65	Condylar breadth (kdl-kdl)	113	–	–	–
68	Mandibular length	103	–	–	98
69	Mentum height (id-gn)	33	–	–	29
72	Total face angle	93°	85°	–	–
73	Medium facial angle	91°	81°	–	–
69	Angulus mandibulae	122°	–	–	118°
47:45	Morphological face index	85.16	–	–	–
48:45	Upper-face index	51.56	55.74	–	–
52:51	Orbital index	88.13 76.19	81.08 75.00	–	–
54:55	Nasal index	40.00	52.00	–	–
8:1	Cranial index x (Garson)	80.23	76.92	76.88	83.14
20:1	Length-height index	56.50	65.38	65.90	66.86
20:8	Breadth-height index	70.42	85.00	85.71	80.42
9:8	Transversal index	65.49	66.43	–	64.34

BIBLIOGRAPHY

Abasa, L. (1929): Ein deformierter Schädel, der bei der Station Melichowskij piwnitschno in Kaukasischen Kreis 1927 gefunden wurde. Antropologiia (Kiev), II, 129-134.

Achmerov, R. (1951): Ufa. Kratkie soobshcheniia Instituta Istorii Material'noi Kul'tury, XL, 132ff.

Aichel, O. (1926): Zur Frage der Erstehung abnormaler Schädelformen. Verhandl. d. Ges. phys. Anthropologie (Stuttgart), I, 16-31.

Aichel, O. (1931-1932): Über künstliche Schädelformation. Verhandlungen d. Ges. phys. Anthropologie (Stuttgart), VI, 76ff.

Akerman, J. (1853): An account of excavation in Anglo-Saxon burial-ground at Harnhall Hill near Salisbury. Archaeologia (London), XXXV, 1-259.

Aleksejev, V. (1954): Palaeoanthropology of the forest tribes of the Northern Altai. Kratkie soobshcheniia AN SSSR. Institut Etnografii, XXI, 63-69.

Ambialet, J. (1893): La déformation artificielle de la tête toulousaine. Thesis, Toulouse.

Ambialet, J. (1893): L'encéphale dans les crânes déformés du Toulousain. L'Anthropologie (Paris), IV, 11-27.

Angel, J. (1936): The human remains from Khirokitia. In: Dikaios, P.: Final report on the excavation of a Neolithic settlement in Cyprus on Behalf of the Department of Antiquities. Appendix II, 416-630.

Angel, J. (1961): Neolithic crania from Sotira. In: Diakaios, P.: Sotira. Published by the University Museum, Univ. of Pennsylvania, Philadelphia.

Anfimov, N. (1951): Meoto-sarmatskij mogilnik u Stanicy Ust-Labinskoj. Materialy i issledovaniia po arkheologii SSSR (Moskva), XXIII, 155ff.

Antonucci, M. (1961): Crani deformati d'un antica serie di Chiusi (epoca tardo-romana). Archivio per l'antropologia e l'etnologia, XCI, 77-82.

Anutschin, D. (1887): Über die alten künstlich deformierten Schädel, di innerhalb der Grenzen Russlands gefunden wurde. In: Protokolle der Sitzungen der Anthropologischen Abteilung der Gesellschaft der Freunde der Naturwissenschaften, Anthropologie und Ethnographie (Moskva), XLIX, 367-414 (in Russian).

Anutchin, D. (1892): Sur les crânes anciens artificiellement déformés trouvés en Russie. Compte-rendus des Congrés Internationaux d'Anthropologie et d'Archéologie préhistoire, II sess., Moscow, I, 263-268.

Arcjutov, N. (1936): The Cemetery of Atkarsk (in Russian). Izvestiia Saratovskogo Nizhne-Volzhskogo Instituta, VII, 1-91.

Asil, N. (1949): Eridu, Sumer (Baghdad) V.

Bachráty, A. (1965): Príspevok k problému umelej deformácie lebky. Acta Facultatis Rerum Naturalium Universitatis Comenianae T. X, Fasc. 1, Anthropologia, XX, 201-203.

Baer, K. (1860): Die Makrokephalen im Boden der Krym und Österreichs, vergliechen mit der Bildung-Abweichung, welche Blumenbach Macrocephalus genannt hat. Mémoires de l'Academie Imp. s. Science de St. Petersburg (St. Petersburg), VII Série, II, Nr. 6.

Balan, M. and Boev, P. (1955): Anthropologische Materialen aus dem Nekropol bei Novi Pasar. Ber. d. Archäol. Inst. d. Bulg. Akad. d. Wiss., XX, 347-370.

Barge, J. (1914): Beiträge zur Kenntnis der neiderländischen Anthropologie. Z. für Morph. und Anthrop. (Stuttgart), XVI, 456-526.

Bartucz, L. (1928): A tököli bronzkori sírmező embertani szempontból. Antropologiai füzetek. Anthropologia Hungarica, III, 1-3.

Bartucz, L. (1936): A kiszombori gepida temető koponyái (Die Gepida-Schädel des Gräberfeldes von Kiszombor). Dolgozatok, XII, 178-204.

Bartucz, L. (1938): A szekszárdi hunkori sír csontvázának antropológiai vizsgálata. Dissertationes Pannonicae, II, 10; Laureae Aquincenses, I, 8-19.

Bartucz, L. (1938): A magyar ember. A Magyar Föld—Magyar Faj sorozat. IV. Budapest. Egyetemi Ed.

Bartucz, L. (1939): Fejünk divatja (Schädelmode—Deformierte Schädel). Buvár V, 565-571.

Bartucz, L. (1966): Die prähistorische Trepanation, Funde mit Medizinhistorischen und Paläopathologischen Beziehungen in Ungarn. Palaeopathologia III. Medicina Ed. Budapest.

Basler, A. (1927): Uber den Einflus der Lagerung von Säuglingen auf die bleibende Schädelform. Z. für Morph. und Anthrop. (Stuttgart), XXVI, 225-246.

Battaglia, R. (1942): Indagini sull'età dei resti umani rinvenuti nella caverne e nel castelliére di San Canziano del Timavo. Atti del Museo civico di Storia naturale Trieste, XV, No. 1, 36ff.

Baudouin, M. (1909): Trois cas de déformation toulousaine du crâne, observés sur des sujets trouves dans le Grotte de Jammes à Martiel (Aveyron). Bull. de Soc. franç. d'Hist. de Méd., VIII, 58-68.

Baudouin, M. (1911): La sépulture néolithique de Belleville à Vendrest (Seine et Marne). Paris.

Baudouin, M. (1911): Etude de l'action sur le cerveau de la déformation annulaire du crâne des Gallo-Romains a l'aide des moulage intracraniens. Comptes-Rendus hebdom. L'Acad. Sci., CLIII, 353-355.

Baudouin, M. (1911): Traces d'action humaine sur le crâne vivant due à une coutume spèciale. <u>Archives Provinciales de Chirurgie</u>, XX, 597-607.

Baudouin, M. (1912): Description anatomique des neuf crânes de la station Gallo-Romaine de Chaumes. <u>Bulletin de la Société d'Anthropologie de Paris</u>, 6me série (Paris), III, 321-346.

Bellasi, P. (1962): La deformazione cranica medioevale in Italia. Contributo antropologico allo studio del problema delle invasioni barbariche. <u>Rivista di Antropologia</u>, XLIX, 25-81.

Beninger, E. (1929): Germanengräber von Laa a.d. Thaya. N.O. <u>Eiszeit und Urgeschichte</u>, VI, 143-155.

Beninger, E. (1932): Der westogotisch-alanische Zug nach Mitteleuropa. <u>Mannus</u>, LI, 30-73.

Beninger, E. (1934): <u>Die Germanenzeit in Niederösterreich.</u> Wien.

Beninger, E. (1937): <u>Die germanische Bodenfunde in der Slowakei.</u> Reihenberg-Leipzig.

Beninger, E. (1942): Germanen in Burgenland. <u>Germanenerbe</u>, VII, 104-149.

Beninger, E. and Freising, H. (1933): <u>Die germanischen Bodenfunde in Mähren.</u> Reichenburg.

Beninger, E. and Mitscha-Märheim, H. (1970): Das langobardische Gräberfeld von Nikitsch, Burgenland. <u>Wiss. Arbeiten aus dem Burgenland</u>, XLIII, p.34.

Bernshtam, A. (1940): Kenkol'skii mogil'nik arkheologicheskoi ekspeditsii Ermitazha. Leningrad.

Bernshtam, A. (1950): Ocherki po istorii gunnov. Moskva-Leningrad.

Bernshtam, A. (1952): Istoriko-arheologitseskie otserki Centralnogo Tjansanja i Pamiro-Alaja. <u>Materiali i Issledovanija po Arheologii SSSR.</u>, (Moskva), XXVI.

Bertholon, L. (1892): Documents anthropologiques sur les Phéniciens. <u>Bulletin de la Société Anthropologique de Lyon</u> (Lyon), XI, 179-224.

Biasutti, R. (1967): Le Razze e i popoli della terra. UTET, (Torino), II, 523.

Björk, A. (1947): The face in profile. <u>Svensk Tandläkare-Tidskr.</u>, XL, No. 5, Lund.

Blondel, L. (1928): Chronique des découveres archéologiques dans le canton de Genéve en 1927. Epoque barbare. Cimitière du Creau de Genthod, Geneva), VI, 27.

Blovatzkij, V. (1951): Phanagoria (Taman). <u>Materialy i issledovaniia po arkheologii SSSR</u>, XIX, 198-200.

Blumenbach, J. (1790): Decas prima collectionis suae craniorum diversarum gentium. Göttingen. Asiatae macrocephali.

Blumenbach, J. (1928): Nova pentas collectionis suae craniorum diversarum gentium tanquam complementum priorum decadum. Göttingen.

Blumenbach, J. (1833): Göttingische gelehrte Anzeigen. Göttingen.

Boas, F. (1924): Bemerkungen über die Anthropometrie der Armenier. Z. für Ethnologie, LVI, 72-82.

Bobij, V. (1957): Iskustvenno deformirovannije tserepa, naudennije pri raskonkah v Krimu. Trudy kaf. norm. Anat. i. Embr. Simferopol.

Boev, P. (1957): Verhu iskustvenite deformacij na glabata. Izvestija na Inst. po Morf. (Sofia), II.

Boev, P. (1957): Protobulgarische künstlich deformierte Schädel. Homo, VIII, No. 3.

Boev, P. (1957): Uber die künstlichen Deformierung des Kopfes. Ber. d. Morph. Inst. d. Bulg. Akad. d. Wiss., II, 263-290 (in Bulgarian).

Boev, P. (1957-59): Protobulgarische künstlich deformierte Schädel. Acta Arch. Hung., X, 155-158.

Bóna, I. (1960): A soponyai germán temető. Alba Regia, I, 165-166.

Bóna, I. (1971): A népvándorlás kora Fejér megyében. Fejér megye története az őskortól a honfoglálslasig, V, 1-94.

Bolta, L. (1968): Rifnik. Prazdogovinska in poznoaticna naselbina in poznoaticno grobisce. Celjski Zbornik, XIV, 209-225.

Borovansky, L. (1936): Pohlavní rozdíly na lebce cloveka. Praha.

Bouffard, P. (1945): Nécropolis burgundes de la Suisse. Genève.

Brandenburg, N. (1899): Emchicha Cemetery (in Russian). Trudy XI, Arch. Sezda Kiev, I, 151ff.

Bräss, M. (1887): Beiträge zur Kenntnis der künstlichen Schädelverbindungen. Mitt. d. Ver. Erdk. Leipzig. Jg., 1886, 131-180.

Brizio, E. (1888): Casalechhio di Reno. Scoperta di due sepolcri antici chi presso l'abitato. Atti della Regia Accademia dei Lincei, Ser. IV, Parte II, Notizie degli Scavi, (Roma), IV, 721-22.

Broca, P. (1864): Sur l'état des crânes et des squelettes dans les anciennes sépultures. Bulletin de la Société d'Anthropologie de Paris, V, 642-653.

Broca, P. (1864): Description du crâne de Voiteur. Bulletin de la Société d'Anthropologie de Paris (Paris), V, 385-392.

Broca, P. (1872): Sur la déformation Toulousaine de crâne. Paris.

Broca, P. (1873): Marche des Cimmériens Macrocéphales. Bulletin de la Société d'Anthropologie de Paris.

Broeck, A. (1916): Zur Frage der willkürlichen Beeinflussung der kindlichen Schädelform. Korr. Bl. Dt. Ges. für Anthrop. und Ethnol. und Urgeschichte (Braunschweig), XLVII, 68-70.

Buchholz, H. and Karageorghis, V. (1971): Altägäis und Altkypros. Verlag Ernst Wasmuth. Tübingen.

Budinský-Kricka, V. (1950): Prehistoricke a ranodejinne nalezy v Leviciach. Arch. Rozhl. (Praha), II, 153-158.

Butschkow, H. (1935): Deformierte Schädel aus Mitteldeutschland. Mitteldt. Volkheit (Halle), II, 47-49.

Buxton, L. (1931): Künstlich deformierte Schädel von Cypern. Anthrop. Anzeiger (Stuttgart), VII, 236-240.

Buxton, D. and Rice, T. (1931): Report on the human remains found at Kish. Journal of the Royal Anthrop. Inst., LXI, 57-120.

Canestrini, G. and Moschen, L. (1978): Sopra un cranio deformato, scavato di Piazza Capitaniato a Padova. Atti della Società Veneto-Tridentina di Scienze Naturali, (Padova), VI, 172-179.

Cappieri, M. (1970): The Mesopotamians of the Chalcolithic and Bronze Ages. Field Research projects, No. XII, 33.

Cauvin, J. (1968): Les outilages néolithiques de Byblos et du littoral libanais. Etudes et Documents d'Archéologie, IV, 359. Paris. Librairie d'Amérique et d'Orient. Adrien Maisonneuve.

Cervinka, I. (1936): Germani na Morave. Anthropologie (Prague), XIV, 107-146.

Chantre, E. (1882): Photographie d'un crâne macrocephale trouve à Marseille. Bulletin de la Société d'Anthropologie de Paris, 3me série, I, 151-152.

Chantre, E. (1886): Recherches anthropologiques dans le Caucase, II, 101ff.; III (1887), 1-47. Bulletin de la Société d'Anthropologie de Paris, 3me série, XI, 198-221.

Chantre, E. (1894): Crâne de la nécropole de Sidon. Bull. Soc. Anthrop. Lyon, XIII.

Chantre, E. (1895): Recherches anthropologiques dans l'Asie Occidentale (Lyon), 68-69; 130.

Chleborad, M. (1914): Archeologicke nalezy okresu bucovickeho v leteh 1912 a 1913. Casopis Morav. Mus. Brno, XIV, 272-282.

Chochol, J. (1969): Ein Küntlich deformierte Kinderschädel aus der Zeit der Völkerwanderung. Fundort Luzec nad Vltavou, Bez. Melnik, Böhmen. Anthropologie (Praha), VII/2, 11-17.

Chvojko, B. (1901): Chernjahov Cemetery (in Russian). Zapiski imp. russk. arkh. obshchestva, XII, 181-205.

Contenson, H. (1965): Remarque sur la sédentarisation au Proche Orient. Berliner Z. für Vor- und Frühgeschichte, XIV, 207-240.

Coon, C. (1949): The Eridu crania, a preliminary report. Sumer (Baghdad), V, 103-106.

Couloma, M. (1931): Considérations générales sur les déformations craniennes et la bathrocéphalie. L'éco medical du nord, XXXV, 253-259.

Critescu, M. (1964): Studiul antropologic al scheletelor dîn secolul al III-1ea e.n. descoperite la Pogorasti (raionul Botosani, reg. Suceava). Arheologia Moldovei, III (Academia Republicii Populare Romîne filiala Iasi), 229-341.

Davis, J. (1862): Notes on the distortions which present themselves in the crania of the Ancient Britons. Natural History Review (London), 290-297.

Davis, J. (1865): On the importance of a due estimate of the different modes and degrees of deformation of the skull in the study of craniology. Stockholm

Davis, J. (1867): Über makrokephale Schädel und über die weibliche Schädelform. Arch. Anthr. (Braunschweig), II, 17-27.

Davis, J. and Thurnam, J. (1856-1865): Crania Britannica (London), II.

Dawson, W. (1927): Artificial deformation of the skull. Lancet, 1376.

Debetz, G. (1948): Paleoantropologiia SSSR. Trudy Instituta etnografii AN SSSR.

Delisle, F. (1889): Sur les déformations artificielles du crâne dans les Deux-Sèvres et la Haute-Garonne. Bulletin de la Société d'Anthropologie de Paris, Sér. III, XIII, 649-659.

Delisle, F. (1902): Les déformations artificielles du crâne en France. Carte de leur distribution. Bulletin de la Société d'Anthropologie de Paris, 5me série, III, 111-167.

Dembo, A. and Imbelloni, J. (1938): Deformaciones intencionales del cuerpo humano de caracter etnico, III. Humanior.

Deshayes, J. (1969): Les civilisations de l'Orient ancien. Paris. Arthaud.

Diaconu, G. (1965): Tirgsor necropola dîn secole III-IV e.n. Bucuresti. Akad.

Dikaios, P. (1953): Khirokitia. Final report on the excavation of a neolithic settlement in Cyprus on behalf of the Department of Antiquities, Oxford, 1936-1946.

Dikaios, P. and Stewart, J. (1962): The Swedish Cyprus Expedition. Vol. IV. The Stone Age and the Early Bronze Age in Cyprus.

Dillenius, J. (1912): Das Scheitelbein unter dem Einfluss des fronto-occipitalen Schädeldeformation. Arch. Anthrop. XXXIX, N.F., 113-138.

Dingwall, J. (1931): Artificial cranial deformation. John Bale Sons and Danielsson. London.

Dombay, J. (1956): Der gotische Grabfund von Domolospuszta. A Janus Pannonius Múzeum Évkönyve, Pécs, 103-130.

Donici, A. (1931): Déformation crânienne en Bessarabie. Nancy.

Drost, D. (1955): Die Skelettfunde von Ingersleben. Altthüringien (Weimar), I, 265-272.

Dubois de Montpéreaux, F. (1832): Voyage autour du Caucase. Vol. V. Paris.

Dunajevskaja, T. (1963): Vliianie iskusstvennoi deformatsii na formu golovy u turkmen. Voprosy antropologii, XV.

Ecker, A. (1866): Skelet eines Makrokephalus in einem fränkischen Todtenfelde. Arch. Anthrop., (Braunschweig), 75-79.

Efimenko, P. and Sovkopljas, I. (1954): Deformacija golovi. Sovjetskaia Arheologiia, XIX, 25ff.

Ehgartner, W. (1953): Zur Anthropologie des Langobardenschädels von Hobersdorf, NO. In: Mitscha-Märheim, H.: Neue Bodenfunde zur Geschichte der Langobarden und Slawen in österreichischen Donauraum. Carinthia, I, 779-780.

Ehrich, R. (1947): Occipital flattening among the Dinarics. Amer. J. Phys. Anthrop., N.S., VI, 181-186.

Eisley, L. (1944): An extreme case of scaphocephaly from a Mound Burial near Troy. Trans. Kansas Acad. Sci. (Kansas), XLVII, 241-235.

Ellerbroeck, N. (1905): Die Scaphokephalen der Göttinger Schädelsammlungen. Med. Diss. Göttingen.

Elsässer, K, (1906): Zur Entstehung von Brachy- und Dolichokephalie durch willkürliche Beeinflussung des kindlichen Schädels. Zentralblatt d. Gynäkol., XXX, 422-424.

Esker, A. (1866): Skelet eines Makrokephalus in einem fränkischen Todtenfelde. Arch. Anthrop. (Braunschweig), I, 75-79.

Ewing, J. (1950): Hyperbrachykephaly as influenced by cultural conditioning. Papers of the Peabody Museum of American Archaeology and Ethnology (Cambridge, Mass.), XXIII, 2. Harvard University.

Falkenburger, F. (1913): Diagraphische Untersuchungen an normalen und deformierten Rassenschädeln. Arch. Anthrop., N.F. (Braunschweig), XII., 81-96.

Falkenburger, F. (1938): Recherches anthropologiques sur la déformation artificielle du crâne. Journal de la Soc. des Américanistes., XXX, facs. 1.

Falkenburger, F. (1938): Sur la déformation, à propos du crâne de Natchez. L'Anthropologie (Paris), XLVIII, 438-441.

Fallot, J. (1881): Note sur une crâne deformée, trouvée à Marseille. Bulletin de la Société d'Anthropologie de Paris, 3me série, IV, 807-812.

Farkas, Gy.(1973): Macrocephalic and "Avar period" mongoloid anthropological finds from Woiwodina. Acta Biologica Szeged, XIX, 1-4, 203-211.

Farkas, Gy. and Lipták, P. (1971): A Tápé környéki leletek értékelése (Evaluation of the finds from the outskirts of Tápé). In: Juhász, A. (edit.): Tápé története és néprajza, 163-167.

Ferembach, D. (1959): Le peuplement du Proche-Orient au Chalcholithique et au Bronze ancient. Israel Exploration Journal (Jerusalem), IX, 221-228.

Field, H. (1948): Head deformation in the Near East. Man (London), XLVIII, No. 145.

Field, H. (1953): Contributions to the anthropology of the Caucasus. Papers of the Peabody Museum of American Archaeology and Ethnology, XLVIII, No. 1, 106-108 (Cambridge, Mass.). Harvard University.

Firstejn, B. (1970): Iskustvenno deformarovannyje cherepa. Voprosy etnogeneza sarmatov po dannym kraniologii. Akademia Nauk SSSR. Institut Etnografia i N. Mikulo-Maklaja. Izdat. Nauka. Leningrad.

Fitzinger, L. (1851): Über Awarenschädel. Sitzungsberichte der Kais. Akademie der Wissenschaften (Wien), VII, 270-281.

Fitzinger, L. (1853): Über die Schädel der Awaren (Inbesondere über sie seither in Osterreich aufgefundenen). Denkschriften des Mathem. naturw. Klasse der Kaiserlichen Akademie der Wissenschaften (Wien), V.

Florschütz, G. (1934): Die vorgeschichtlichen Sammlungen des Gothaer Heimatsmuseum. Gotha.

Flower, W. (1890): Exhibition of an artificially deformed skull from Mallicolo. J. Anthrop Inst., XIX, 52.

Folmer, H. (1897): Een geval van sphenolordese ten gevolge van kunstmatige schedelmisvorming. Amsterdam.

Folmer, H. (1898): La déformation artificielle du crâne chez les enfants nouveau-nes. Gazette médicale de Paris (Paris), 2e série, 600-602; 624-625.

Franz, L. (1933): Der Germanenfriedhof von Tschelakowitz. Sudentendeutsches Jahrbuch., XLI, 36-44.

Frassetto, F. (1918): Lezioni di antropologia, II, Parte I (Milano), 341-353.

Fridolin, J. (1909): Die deformierten Schädel die in Alutsch auf der Krim gefunden werden sind. Jahrbuch d. russ. Anthropologischen Gesellschaft III (in Russian).

Fritsch, G. (1875): Die Ausgrabungen von Samthawro und Kertsch. Verhandlungen der Berliner Gesellschaft für Anthropologie, Ethnologie und Urgeschichte (Berlin), 152-154.

Fürst, C. (1930): Zur Anthropologie der prähistorischen Griechen.

Fürst, C. (1931): Zur Kenntnis der Anthropologie der prehistorischen Bevölkerung der Insel Cypern. Lunds Un. Arkr., N.F., Adv. II, Bd. 29.6, et. Kungsl. Fysiograf. sälsk. Handlingar. N.F., Bd. XLIV, 6 (Lund).

Fürst, K. (1909): Das Skelett von Viste auf Jäderen. Ein Fall von Scaphokephalie aus der älteren Steinzeit. Videns Selsk. Skr. Mathem. Nat., Kl. I.

Gáspár, J. (1931): Gepidengräber aus Ungarn. Mitt. d. Anthrop. Ges. in Wien, LXI, 289ff.

Gáspár, J., (1932): Gepidengräber aus Ungarn. Mitteilungen der Anthropologischen Abteilung des Anatomischen Instituts an der Universität Szeged, 285-291.

Generisch, G. (1903): A bölcső hatása a koponya fejlődésére (Die Einwirkung der Wiege auf die Schädelentwicklung). Természettud. Közlemények, XXXV, 640.

Gerhardt, K. (1939): Eine Mongolin in germanischen Thüringen des 7. Jhdts. Gothaisches Tageblatt vom 16.iii.1939.

Gerhardt, K. (1965): Zwei künstlich deformierte Schädel aus Merowingischen Reihengräbern im Donaubogen bei Regensburg. Beitr. z. Oberpfalzforschung, I, 13-15.

Gerhardt, K. (1965?): Zwei merowingzeitliche deformierte Schädel in ihrer anthropologischen und ethnologischen Problematik. 8. Tagung der deutschen Gesellschaft für Anthropologie, 237-239.

Geyer, E. (1932): Wiener Grabfunde au der Zeit des untergehende römischen Limes. Wiener Prähistorische Zeitschrift, XIX.

Ghirshman, R. (1948): Les Chionites-Hephtalites. Mém. Déleg. francaise en Afganistan, XIII. Cairo.

Giltshenko, V. (1890): Material on the Anthropology of the Caucasus. Trudy Institut Antropologii i Etnografii USSR. Academy of Sciences (Leningrad), Vol. XVI, No. 2.

Gindre, P. and Moretin, L. (1864): Crâne extraordinairement déformé, trouvé à Voiteur (Jura). Bulletin de la Société d'Anthropologie de Paris, V, 383-384.

Ginzburg, V. (1937): Gornye tadzhiki. Materialy po antropologii tadzhikov Karategina i Darbaza. Moskva-Leningrad.

Ginzburg, V. (1950): Materialy k paleoantropologii vostochnykh raionov srednei Azii. Kratkie Soobssheniia Instituta Etnografii, XI.

Ginzburg, V. (1954): Materialy k antropologii drevnego naseleniia iuzhnogo Kazakhstana. Sovjetskaia Arheologiia (Moskva-Leningrad), XXI, 379-394.

Ginzburg, V. (1956): Drevnee naselenie vostochnykh i tsentral'nykh raionov Kazakhskoi SSR po antropologicheskim dannym. Trudy Instituta Etnografii N.S., XXXIII. Moskva.

Ginzburg, V. (1956): Materialy k antropologii drevnego naseleniia Ferganskoi doliny. Trudy Kirgizkoi arkheo-etnograficheskoi ekspeditsii. (Moskva), I, 85-86.

Ginzburg, V. and Zirov, E. (1949): Antropologicheskie materialy iz Kenkol'skogo katakombnogo mogil'nika v doline r. Talas, Kirgizkoi SSR. Sbornik Muzeia Antropologii i Etnografii (Moskva-Leningrad), X, 213-265.

Giuffrida-Ruggeri, V. (1906): Crânes européens déformés. Revue de l'Ecole d'Anthropologie de Paris, 6me année (Paris), September 1906, 316-324.

Gosse, H. (1853): Suite à la Notice cimetières trouvés, soit en Savoie, soit dans le canton Genève. Mémoires de la Soc. d'Hist. et d'Arch. de Genève, 1-7.

Gosse, H. (1855): Notice sur d'anciens cimetières. Mém. de la Soc. d'Hist. et d'Arch. de Genève, IX.

Gosse, L. (1855): Essai sur les déformations artificielles du crâne (Paris), 43.

Gosse, L. (1855): Essai sur les déformations artificielles du crâne. Annales d'Hygène publique et de Médicine Légale, 2me serie (Paris), III, 317-393 and IV, 5-88.

Grjaznov, M. (1928): Fürstengräber im Altaigebiet. Wiener Prähistorische Zeitschrift, XV, 120-123.

Grjaznov, M. (1947): Raboty altaiskoi ekspeditsii. Kratkie soobshcheniia Instituta istorii material'noi kul'tury. Raskopi altaiskoi ekspeditsii na Blizhnik (Elbanakh), 111.

Greenwell, W. (1877): British Barrows. London.

Hamy, E. (1868): Sur deux nouveaux cas de déformations crâniennes observés à Paris. Bulletin de la Société d'Anthropologie de Paris, III, 301-303.

Hancar, F. (1937): Mittelbronzezeitliche Katakombengräber im Manytschtal und bei Elista. Tallgren-Festschrift, SMYA, XLV, 75ff.

Hankó, I. (1968): Koranépvándorláskori gazdag női sír embertani anyagának ismertetése (The examination of a rich Female Find by Regöly from the Early Migration Period). Anthropologiai Közlemények, XII, 3-4, 117-123.

Hankó, I. and Kiszely, I. (1973): Artificially deformed male skull of the Early Migration Period from Tamási-Adorjánpuszta (in Hungarian). Szekszárdi Múzeum Évkönyve, II, 67-84.

Haruzin, A. (?): Les Anciens Tombs du Gurzuf et Gugush.

Hatt, G. (1915): Artificial moulding of the infant head among the Scandinavian Lapps. Amer. Anthrop., XVII, 244-256.

Heikel, H. (1918): Altertümer aus dem Tale des Talas in Turkestan. Trav. ethnogr. de la Soc. finno-ougrienne, (Helsinki), VII.

Heikel, A. (1894): Excavation du Tsuvash. Antiquités de la Sibérie occidentale, XXI. Materialy i issledovaniia po arkheologii SSSR (Moskva), XXXV, 192.

Helmuth, H. (1970): Über den Bau des menschlichen Schädels bei künstlicher Deformation. Z. Morph. und Anthrop., LXII, 1, 30-49.

Helmuth, H. (1973): Zwei küntlich deformierte Schädel aus Altenerding. 54. Bericht der Römisch-Germanischen Kommission (Darmstadt), 304-317.

Henschen Folke (1966): Der Menschliche Schädel in der Kulturgeschichte. Springer Verlag. Berlin-Heidelberg.

Hervé, G. (1901): Crâne macrocéphale de Saint-Prex. Bulletin de la Société d'Anthropologie de Paris, 5me serie, II, 583-585.

Heukemes, B., Hoepke, H. and Kindler, W. (1956): Künstliche Schädelmissbildung ungewöhnlicher Art aus eunem fränkischen Grabfund des 7. Jh. bei Heidelberg, (Ruperto-Carola), VIII, Bd. XIX. Heidelberg.

His, W. and Rütimeyer, L. (1864): Crania Helvetica. Basel-Genf.

Hoepke, H. (1959): Ein missbildeter Schädel aus einem fränkischen Grab bei Heidelberg-Dossenheim. Morphologisches Jahrbuch, (IC, H.4, 691-709.

Hoffmann, R. (1939): Spätgermanische Grabfunde von Phöben, Kreis Zauch-Belzig. Mannus (Leipzig), XXXI, 295-313.

Holter, F. (1925): Das Gräerfeld bei Obermöllern aus der Zeit des alten Thüringen. Jhschr. f. mitteldt. Vorgeschichte, XII, H.1, 1-114.

Imbelloni, J. (1925): Numero de los tipos fundamentales cé los que debun referisce les deformaciones craneanas. Buenos Aires.

Imbelloni, J. (1930): Die Arten der künstlichen Schädeldeformation. Anthropos, XXV, 801-830.

Imbelloni, J. (1935): Uber Formen, Wesen und Methoden der absichtlichen Deformation. Z. für Morph. und Anthrop., XXXIII, 164-189.

Istrati, C. (1900): Sur les crânes trouvés á Constantza (Kustenjé) Dobsodja. Bulletin de la Société des Sciences de Boucarest (Bucareşti), IX, 613-319.

Ivanovskij, A. (1891): Cherepa iz mogil'nikov Ossetii. Izvestiia obshchestva liubitelei estestvoznaniia, antropolgii i etnografii, XXI. Trudy antropologicheskeva otdela, XIII, No. 5. Moskva.

Jarho, A. (1933): Türkmeni Horezma i Severnava Kavkaza. Antropologicheskii zhurnal. Nos. I-II, 70-119.

Jarho, A. (1953): Antropologicheskii sostav turetskikh narodnostei Srednei Azii. Antropologicheskii zhurnal, III, 2-28.

Jazuta, K. (1925): Uber künstliche deformierte Schädel aus Südrussland. Nachrichten des staatlichen Don-Universität, Tom. V, (Rostov-on-Don) (in Russian).

Javorskij, I. (1895): Antropologitsheskii i etnografitsheskii Ocherki turkmeni. Odessa.

Jelinek, J. (1958): Ein künstlich deformierte Kinderschädel aus der Zeit der Völkerwanderung. Casopis Moravského Muzea, XLIII, 181-182.

Jelinek, J. (1960): Vier deformierte Schädel aus der Völkerwanderungszeit aus Südmähren. Casopis Moravského Muzea, XLV, 251-264.

Jungwirth, J. and Kiszely, I. (in the press): Anthropologische Bearbeitung des burgstaller Kinderskeletts mit deformiertem Schädel.

Karageorghis, V. (1968): Chypre. Editions Nagel. Genève-Paris-München.

Karageorghis, V. (1976): Kition. Mycenean and Phoenician Discoveries in Cyprus. Thames and Hudson. London.

Katona, F. (1969): Az agy felfedezése. Gondolat Ed. Budapest.

Katona, F. (1974): Embérrévalás. Gondolat Ed. Budapest.

Kaufmann, H. (1955): Altthüringer Gräber auf Sidlungsstätte in Ingersleben, Kr. Erfurt. Altthüringen (Weimar), I, 1953-1954, 255-264.

Keim, J. (1928): Ausgrabungen und Funde von Streubing Umgebung. Jahresbericht d. Hist. Ver. f. Streubing und Ungebung, XXXI, Straubing.

Keith, A. (1929): Human skulls from Ancient Cemeteries in the Tarim Basin. J. Anthrop. Inst. of Great Britain, LIX, 149-180.

Khudayberdiev, D. (1968): The cranial index of the Türkmens. VIIme Congres Anthropologique et Ethnologique du Moscou, 1964. Izdat. Nauk. SSSR. Moskva.

Kindler, W. (1957): Röntgenologische Untersuchungen eines künstlich deformierten Schädels aus der Völkerwanderungszeit. Fortschritte auf dem Gebiete der Röntgenstrahlen und der Nuklearmedizin (Stuttgart), LXXXVII, H.2, 185-190.

Kindler, W. (1957): Die künstliche Schädeldeformierung. Kult- und Modelbrauch seit über fünf Jahrtausenden. Umschau LVII (Frankfurt am Main), 567-569.

Kindler, W. (1958): Vorrichtungen zur künstlichen Schädeldeformierung im Dienst von Kultur und Schönheit im Laufe der Jahrtausende. Med. Kosmetik, VII, 33-39.

Kindler, W. (1963): Künstliche Schädeldeformierung im Laufe der Jahrtausende. Panorama. Mai.

Kiseljev, S. (1951): Drevniia istoriia iuzhnoi Sibiri. Moskva.

Kiszely, I. (1969): Sirok, csontok, emberek (Graves, bones, men), Gondolat Ed. Budapest. 2nd edition, 1976.

Kiszely, I. (1969): Anthropologische Untersuchung der frühvölkerwanderungszeitlichen Skelettfunde mit künstlich deformierte Schädeln von Letkés. Mitt. des Arch. Inst. des Ung. Akademie der Wissenschaften (Budapest), II, 103-117.

Kiszely, I. (1969): Le caratteristiche antropologiche delle tombe longobarde di di Fiesole. Accademia Toscana di Scienze e Lettere "La Columbaria" (Firenze), XXXV, 77-100.

Kiszely, I. (1970): Short anthropological characterization of the Langobard Age Cemetery at Kranj. Glasnik Antropoloskog Drustva Jugoslavije. Sveska (Beograd), VII, 65-79.

Kiszely, I. (1971): Anthropologische Untersuchung der Frühvölkerwanderungszeitlichen Skelettfunde mit künstlich deformierten Schädeln von Letkés. Mitt. des Arch. Inst. der Ung. Akademie der Wissenschaften (Budapest), II, 103-117.

Kiszely, I. (1972): Der deformierte Schädel im Grabfund von Kesztölc. Mitt. des Arch. Inst. der Ung. Akademie der Wissenschaften (Budapest), III, 123-127.

Kiszely, I. (1973): Torzított koponyájú sírlelet rekonstruált arca. Somogyi Múzeumok Közleményei, I, 299-301.

Kiszely, I. (1976): A Langobard ethnikum anthropológiája. Dissertation. Budapest Akademie d. Wissenschaften.

Kiszely, I. (1976): Artificial skull-deformations in Europe of the early Migration Period; as they had been valued previously and as they are considered today. Acta Congressus Internationalis XXIV, Historiae Artis Medicinae, 25-31, August 1974 (Budapest), 1309-1315.

Kiszely, I. (1976): Anthropologische Bearbeitung der prälangobardischen Gräber von Soponya. Mitt. des Arch. Inst. der Ung. Akademie der Wissenschaften (Budapest), VI, 125-131.

Kiszely, I. (1978): Rassengeschichte von Ungarn. In: Schwidetzky, I. (ed.): Rassengeschichte der Menschheit, V, 104-137. Oldenburg Verlag. München-Wien.

Kiszely, I. and Hankó, I. (1971-1972): Mesterségesen deformált koranépvándorláskori férifikoponya Tamási-Adorjánpusztáról. A Szekszárdi Balogh Adám Múzeum Evkönyve (Szekszárd), 67-84.

Kiszely-Hankó, I. (1974): A Brief anthropological characterization of three artifically deformed skulls from Sweden. Ossa (Stockholm), I, 38-50.

Klaatsch, H. (1913): Morphologische Studien zur Rassendiagnostik der Turfanschädel. Abh. Preuss. Akad. phys-mathem. Kl., (Berlin), 1912, III.

Kohler, G. (1901): Die künstliche Deformation des Schädels. Erlangen. Phil. Diss. 1898.

Körber, E. (1957): Abrazion und Artukulationsbewegung. Deutsch. Zahnarztl. Zeitschrift, XII, 1486-1490.

Kucharenko, J. (1954): Csernjahov. Sovietskaia Arkheologiia, XIX, 119ff.

Kucharenko, J. (1954): K voprosu o slaviano-skifskikh i slaviano-sarmatskikh otnosheniiakh. Sovietskaia Arkheologiia, XIX, 111ff.

Kudrnac, J. (1952): Pohrebiste z doby stehovaní národu v Klucove. Archeologické Rozhledy, IV, 109-112.

Kurth, G. (1955): Vorbericht über anthropologische Beobachtung bei den Jerichograbung 1955. Homo, VI, 145-156.

Kurth, G. (1958): Zur Stellung der neolithischen Menschenreste von Khirokitia aud Cypern. Homo, IX, 20-31.

Kurth, G. (1958): Jericho und Byblos. Homo, VIII, 197-207.

Kurth, G. (1967): Erste Ergebnisse und Probleme bei der Untersuchung des Jerichomaterials. Homo, XIX, 79-81.

Kurth, G. (1969): Bevölkerungsbewegung im östlichen Mittelmeerraum. Archeologia Viva, III.

Kurth, G. (1973): "Neolithische" Menschenreste des weiteren Nahostraums. In: Fundamenta. Monographien zur Urgeschichte. Teil VIIIa. Anthropologie. Teil I. Böhlau. Köln.

Lagneau, G. (1864): Lecture a l'occasion du crâne de Voiteur. Bulletin de la Société d'Anthropologie de Paris, VI, 421-427.

Lagneau, G. (1879): De déformations céphaliques en France. Gazette hebdomadaire de Médicine et Chirurgie, 2me série, XVI, 72-75; 89-92.

Lagotala, H. (1921): Au sujet de quelques crânes déformés, provenant du dolmen de Guizy. Comptes-rendus de l'Association française pour l'Avancement des Sciences (Rouen), 784-787.

Lebzelter, V. (1935): Zur Frage der Veränderung der deutschen Schädelform. Zeitschrift für Rassenkunde, I, 90-117.

Lebzelter, V. and Thalmann, G. (1935): Über die Rassengliederung der Langobarden. Forschungen und Fortschritte, XI, No. 25, 318-319.

Lecourtois, E. (1869): Sur la forme et le developement du crâne chez les nouveaunés. Bulletin de la Société d'Anthropologie de Paris, Sér. 2, IV, 820-824.

Lenhossék, J. (1877): Description 'd'un crâne macrocéphale déformé et d'un crâne de l'époque barbare en Hongrie. Congrès international d'Anthrop. et d'Archéol. préhistorique. Budapest.

Lenhossék, J. (1878): Des déformations artificielles du crânes en générale. Budapest.

Lenhossék, J. (1978): Die künstlichen Schädelverbindungen im allgemeinen und zwei künstlich vervildete makrokephale Schädel aus Ungarn sowie ein Schädel aus der Barbarenzeit Ungarns. Budapest. Neudruck Wien. 1881.

Lenhossék, J. (1878): Über künstlich deformierte Schädel im allgemeinen und im besonderen über je einen makrokephalen Schädel solcheart aus Csongrád und Székelyudvarhely, bzw. einen aus der Barbarenzeit aus Alcsuth (Budapest), 1-127.

Lenhossék, J. (1882): A szeged-öthalmi ásatásokról és egy Ó-Szőnyről kiasott mesterségesen eltorzított makrokephal koponyáról. Magyar Tudományos Akadémia Könyvkiadó Hivatala (Budapest), 141.

Lenhossék, J. (1886): Die Ausgrabungen zu Szeged-Öthalom in Ungarn, namentlich die in den dortigen urmagyarischen, altrömischen und keltischen Gräbern aufgefundene Skelette, darunter ein sphenocephaler und katarrhiner hyperchamaecephaler Schädel, ferner ein dritter und vierter künstlich verbildeter makrocephaler Schädel aus Ó-Szőny und Pancsova in Ungarn. Wien.

Levin, M. (1947): Deformaciia golobi i türkmeni. Sovietskaia Etnografiia, VI-VII, 184-190.

Lippert, A. (1968): Ein Gräberfeld des Völkerwanderungszeit bei Grafenwörth p.B. Tulln. NO. Mitt. der Anthrop. Ges. in Wien, XCVIII, 35-48.

Lipták, P. (1961): Germanische Skelettreste von Hács-Béndekpuszta aus dem 5. Jahrhundert U. Z. Acta Archeologica (Budapest), XIII, 231-246.

Lloyd, S. (1947): Eridu, Sumer (Baghdad), III, No. 2, 84-95.

Lloyd, S. and Safar, F. (1947-1948): A preliminary communication on the Second Season's Excavations 1947-1948, Eridu, Sumer (Baghdad), IV, 115-125.

Lobligeois, C. (1869): Déformation oblique de la tête chez les enfants nouveau-nés. Gazette hebdomadaire de Médicine et Chirurgie, 2me Série, VI, 728-729.

Lorenzová, A. (1958): Pathologische und artefizielle Schädeldeformation aus der Völkerwanderungszeit. Spisy vydàvane prirodovedecké fakulty Masarikovy University, Brno, CCCXCVII, 371-387.

Lorenzová, A. (1959): Umele deformovaná lebka z Vicemilic. Časopis Moravskeho musea, Scientiae naturales, XLIV, 203-210.

Lorenzová, A. (1960): Umele deformované lebky z Velatic. Spisy prirodovedecké fakulty Masarikovy University, Brno, CCCCXVI, 333-371.

Lorenzová, A. (1961): Dékla zivota abyvartel Jizni Moravy v protohistorickýh sobáh slovanských. Anthropos (Brno), XIV, 157-166.

Lorenzová, A. (1963): Studie deformovaných lebek z Moravy. Dissertation. Brno, kveten Antropologicky Ustav. UJEP.

Lorenzová, A. (1963): Pathologische und Artefizielle Schädeldeformationen aus der Völkerwanderungszeit. Brno. Masarikovy University.

Lorenzová, A. (1964): Deformierte Schädel aus Náklo und ein weiterer neuer Skelettfund mit deformiertem Schädel aus Sedlesovice. Sbornik III. Karlu Tihelkovi. Archeologicky Ustav CSAV (Brno), 156-161.

Lorenzová, A., Pospísil, M. and Kalus, L. (1957): Novy nález kostry s deformovanou lebkou z. Vacenovic. Studie krajskeho musea v Gottwaldowe, Spolecenské vedy, XIV, 22-23.

Loritz, I. (1915): Altbulgarische Schädel. Dissertation. München.

Loritz, I. (1915): Über die Herkunft des südbulgarischen Dolichocephalus. Correspondbl. Anthr. Ges. München, 21-26.

Lortet, L. (1884): Cause des déformations que présentent les crânes des Syro-Phéniciens. Bull. de la Société Anthropologique de Lyon (Lyon), III, 30-40.

Luckevic, I. (1952): The Cemetery at Neshtsheretovo-Neshtsherove (in Russian). Arheologiia (Kiev), 136-141.

Lunier, R. (1832): Recherches sur quelques déformations crâniennes observées dans le départment des Deux-Sèvres Paris.

Luschan, F. (1886): Wandervölker Kleinasiens. Verhandlungen der Berliner Gesellschaft für Anthropologie, Ethnologie und Urgeschichte (Berlin, 167-171.

Maceda, M. (1972): Artificial cranial deformation: its practice in the past in some Bisayan Islands in the Philippines. In: Proceedings of the First Regional Seminar on South-east Asian Prehistory and Archeology, Manila (National Museum of the Philippines), 27-36.

Malafa, R. (1934): Kostrové pozustatky pohrebiste staroslovenskeho ve Starém Meste u Uherskeho Hradiste. Sbornik Velahradiste, I, 3-16.

Malconian, B. and Schaepelynck, J. (1947): Sur une déformation crânienne au Liban. Bulletin de la Société d'Anthropologie de Paris, 9me Série, VIII,

Malý, J. (1935): Umele deformovane lebky z Celakovic u Prahy. Anthropologie (Praha), XIII, 1-2, 37-53.

Malý, J. (1936): Lebky z II. hribu ve Strazich (Praha), IX, 27-28.

Manouvrier, L. (1889): Discussion sur les déformations du crâne. Bulletin de la Société d'Anthropologie de Paris, 3me Série, XIII, 659-661.

Martin, R. (1928): Lehrbuch der Anthropologie. Fischer Verlag, Jena. 2nd edition.

Matiegka, J. (1894): Umele deformovaná lebka z Budyne v Čechák. Rospravéch II. tr. Ceské Akademie.

Matiegka, J. (1927): Deformace, mutilace a okraslovani lidskeho tela. Anthropologie, Praha.

McNeil, R. and Newton, G. (1965): Cranial Base Morphology in Association with International Cranial Vault Deformation. Amer. J. Phys. Anthrop., XXIII, 241-253.

Meigs, J. (1859): Description of a deformed fragmentary human skull, found in an ancient quarry-cave at Jerusalem. Philadelphia.

Melconiai, B. and Schaepeynick, J. (1947): Sur une déformation crânienne observée au Liban. Bulletin de la Société d'Anthropologie de Paris, 8me série, 48-54.

Melnik, E. (1902): The Cemetery at Voronovka (in Russian). Trudy Arch. S'ezda, (Kharkov), XII, 1, 723ff.

Messeri, P. (1955): Aspetti della base in crani calchaqui deformati. Archivio per l'Antropologia e la Etnologia (Firenze), LXXXV, 1-22.

Messeri, P. (1962): Proposta di un metodo per il riconoscimento della deformazione artifiziale del cranio. Rivista di Scienze Preistoriche, XVII, Fasc. 1-4, 223-236.

Meyer, K. (1850): Beschreibung eines bei Kertsch in der Halbinsel Krym aufgefundenen Stirnbeines ein Makrocephalus. J. Müllers Arch. f. Anat. und Phys., 250ff.

Miletič, N. (1970): Arheološka istraživanja ranosrednjovjekovne nekropole u Rakovcanima kod Prijedora, u ovum broju Glasnika. Glasnika Zemaljsko muz. BiH. sv. XXV. Archeologija. Sarajevo.

Miller, V. (1881-1887): Otshenskii etudi, I-III. Moskva.

Miller, V. (1888): Osorukova (Urusbevo). Materialy po Arkeologii Kavkaza, I, 78ff.

Minaeva, T. (1951): Arheologitsheskii pamiatniki na r. Giljac c verchociach Kubani. Materialy i issledovaniia po arkheologii SSSR (Moskva), 273-301.

Minaeva, T. (1927): Progrebeniia s sozzeniiem gor. Pokrovska Uchenii Zapiski Univ., Saratov, VI, 91-127.

Minaeva, T. (1927): Semiglavii Mar. Uchenii Zapiski Univ., Saratov, VI, 119.

Minaeva, T. (1929): Zwei Kurgane aus der Völkerwanderungszeit bei der Station Sipovo. Eurasia Septentrionalis Antiqua (Helsinki), IV.

Miszkiewicz, B. (1935): An artificially deformed skull from Zlota. Przeglad Antrop., XXI, 1396-1405 (in Polish).

Mitscha-Märheim, H. (1953): Neue Bodenfunde zur Geschichte der Langobarden und Slawen in österreichischen Donauraum. Egger Festschrift, II, 355-376.

Mitscha-Märheim, H. (1963): Dunkler Jahrhundertemgoldene Spuren. Die Völkerwanderungszeit in Osterreich. Wien.

Mitscha-Märheim, H. (1966): Das langobardisches Gräberfeld von Steinbrunn und die Völkerwanderungszeitliche Besiedlung des Ortgebietes. Wissenschaftliches Arbeiten aus dem Burgenland, XXXV, Festschrift für Alfons A. Barb (Eisenstadt), 104-114.

Moiberg, G. (1946): The Cemetery at Belbek (in Russian). Sovietskaya Arheologiia, VIII, 115ff.

Moss, M. (1958): The Pathogenesis of Artificial Cranial Deformation. Amer. J. Phys. Anthrop., N.S., XVI, 269-286.

Much, M. (1898): Uber einen Freifhof aus der Lombardenzeit. Correspondenz blatt der deutschen Gesellschaft für Anthropologie, Ethnologie und Urgeschichte, 164-166.

Müller, G. (1936): Zur Anthropologie der Langobarden. Mitt. d. Anthrop. Gesellschaft in Wien, LXVI, 345-355.

Necrasov, O. and Antoniu, S. (1962): Sur un crâne présentant une déformation dite "macrocéphale", découvert à Tatina-Spantov. Annale Stiintifice ale Universitatii Al. I. Cuza, N.S., VIII, No. 1, 115-127.

Necrasov, O. and Botezatu, D. (1967): Studiul Antropologic al unui schelet din perioda Hunica. Studii si Cercetari de Antropologie, Tomul IV, (Bucaresti), 171-174.

Nemeskéri, J. (1944-1945): A gyöngyösapati hunkori sír torzított koponyájának antropológiai vizsgálata. Archeológiai Értesítő, II, Vol. V-VI, 303-312.

Nemeskéri, J. (1952): An anthropological examination on recent macrocephalic finds. Acta Archaeologica Academiae Scient. Hungariae (Budapest), II, 223-233.

Neumann, A. (1965): Spital und Bad des Legionslagers Vindobona. Jahrbuch des Römisch-Germanischen Zentralmuseums Mainz, XII, 99-117.

Neústupný, J. (1936): Prispevky k dobe stehování narodu v karpatské Kotliné, OP, IX. (1930-1935) (Praha), 11-27; 29-32.

Nicolaescu-Plopșor, S. (1961): Anthropologische Befunde über die Skelettreste aus dem Hunnengrab von Dulceanca (Rayon Rosiori). Dacia, V.

Niederle, L. (1892): Die neuentdeckter Gräber von Podbaba und der erste künstlich deformierte prähistorische Schädel aus Böhmen. Mitt. d. Anthrop. Ges. in Wien, XXII, N.F., 1-18.

Niklasson, N. (1929): Gräber der Merowingerzeit in Lützen, Kr. Merseburg. Jschr. f. mitteldt. Vorgesch (Halle), XVII, 67-85.

Oetteking, B. (1924): Declination on the pars basilaris in normal and artificially deformed skulls. Indian Notes and Monographs, XXVII, 1-25.

Orsi, F. (1894): Nuove scoperta nella necropoli del Fusco. Atti della R. Accademia dei Lincei, Anno CCXCI, Ser. V, Vol. II, parte 2. Notizie degli Scavi (Roma), 152.

Orsi, F. (1895): Siracusa. Gli scavi nella necropoli del Fusco a Siracusa, nel Giugno November 3 Dicembre 1893. Atti della R. Accademia dei Lincei, Anno CCXCII, Serie V, Vol. III, parte 2. Notizie degli scavi (Roma), 117.

Oshanin, L. (1925): L'ancienneté millénaire de la dolichocéphalie des Turcomans. Antropologitscheskii Zhurnal (Moskva), XIV, 69-70.

Oshanin, L. (1928): Einige ergänzende Angeben zur Hypothese des skythosarmatischen Ursprungs der Turkmenen. Nachrichten d. mittelasiatischen Komitees in Sachen der Museen, III, Tashkent (in Russian).

Oshanin, L. (1959): Antropologicheskii sostav turkmenskii plemen i etnogeneza turkmenskava naroda. Trudy Iuzno-Turkmenistanskoi Arkheologitsheskoi ekspeditsii, IX, I.

Oshanin, L. (1959): Antropologitsheskii sostav naseleniya Srednei Azii i etnogenez yeye narodov. Yerevan.

Otten, Ch. (1948): Note on the Cemetery of Eridu, Sumer (Baghdad), IV, 125-127.

Ozbek, M. (1974): Etude de la déformation crânienne artificielle chez les Chalcolithiques de Byblos (Liban). Bulletin de la Société d'Anthropologie de Paris, I, 13me Série, 455-481.

Ozbek, M. (1974): A propos des déformations crâniennes artificielles observées au Proche-Orient. Paléorient, II, No. 2, 469-476.

Pacher, M. (1965): Anthropologischer Befund von Wien-Salvatorgasse (longobardisch). In: Neumann, A.: Spital und Bad des Legionarslagers Bindobona. Jahrbuch des Römisch Germanisches Zentralmuseums Mainz, 117-126.

Palliardi, J. (1888): Predhistorické památky mesta Znojma. Casopis Vlasteneckeho spolku Mujeznihov Olomuci, V, 53-58; 150-157.

Pankow, G. (?): Untersuchungen über die Schädelbasisverknickung beim Menschen. Z. menschl. Vererb. Konst., IX, 69-139.

Párducz, M. (1963): Die ethnische Probleme der Hunnenzeit in Ungarn. Studia Arch. I, Budapest. Academic Press.

Pavelcik, J. (1949): Kosterni material z výkopu ve Starem Meste v. 1948. Zprávy Antropologické Spolecnosti Rocnik II, No. 2-4 (Brno), XV, Listopadu, 24-31.

Pfisterer, H. (1961): Schädelbasisveränderungen bei künstlich deformierten Schädeln in röntgenologischer, kraniometrischer und klinischer Sicht. Monatsschrift für Ohrenheilkunde und Laryngo-Rhinologie XCV, Heft 3, 125-135.

Pic, J. (1892): Hroby s kostramy v Podbabe z doby stehovàni národu. Pamatky Arch., XV, 633-656.

Pilaric, G. (1970): Antropoloska Istrazivanja artificijelno deformiranih lubanja iz ranosrednojovjekovne nekropole u Rakovcanima kod prijedora. Gasnika Zemaljskog muzeja BiH, No. XXV. Archeologija (Sarajevo), 179-195. In German: Wiss. Mitt. des Bosnisch-herzegowinischen Landesmuseum, Bd. III, Heft A, Archeologie.

Pittart, E. (1900): Note sur deux crânes macrocephales trouvés dans un tumulus à Kustendje. Bull. Soc. des Sciences de Bucarest, N.S., IX, 620-629.

Pittard, E. (1901): Note sur les deux crânes macrocéphales trouvés dans un tumulus à Constanza (Dobrodja). Bull. Societé des Sc. Bucarest, X, No. 6, 14-19.

Pittard, E. and Donici, A. (1931): Quelques crânes de Roumanie présentant la déformation macrocéphalique. Archives Suisses d'Anthropologie générale, VI, 1, 44-54.

Posta, B. (1905): Archäologische Studien auf russischen Boden, 556.

Poulik, J, (1948-50): Jizni Morava, zeme dávnych slovanu. Brno.

Pruner-Bey, D. (1866): Crânes de Syrie. Bulletin de la Société d'Anthropologie de Paris, 2me série (Paris), I, 564-572.

Rasoumovsky, G. (1830): Quelques vues sur les Alpes de l'Autriche. Isis, der encyclopädische Zeitung von Oken, XXIII, 143-162.

Rathke, F. (1843): Uber die Makrocephali bei Kertsch in der Krimm. Arhiv für Anatomie, Physiologie U.S.W., 142-148.

Rau, P. (1926): Die Hügelgräber römischer Zeit an der unteren Wolga. Mitteilungen des Zentralmuseums d. Aut. Soz. Räte-Republik der Wolgadeutsch. n. I. Pokrovsk.

Rau, P. (1927): Prähistorische Ausgrabungen auf der Steppenseite des deutschen Wolga-gebietes im Jahre 1926. Mitteilungen des Zentralmuseums d. Aut. Soz. Räte-Republik der Wolga-deutschen. II. Pokrovsk.

Regnault, F. (1906): Les terre-cuites grèques de Smyrne. Bulletin de la Société d'Anthropologie de Paris, 5me série, 1900, 467-477.

Regnault, F. (1907): Comment les anciens considéraient les crânes déformés. Comptes-rendus de l'Association francaise pour l'Avancement des Sciences, 36me session. Reims.

Regöly-Mérei, Gy. (1960): Kórbonctani szempontok a sírletetek torzult és torzított koponyáinak vizsgálatakor, különös tekintettel a Domolospusztai leletre. A Janus Pannonius Múzeum Évkönyve, Pécs, 265-284.

Repnikov, N. (1906): Izvestia Imperatorskoi Arkheologiceskoi Kommissii, XIX, 5ff.

Robin, V. (1957): Iskusstvenno fedormirovannie cerepa naidennie pri raskopkach v Krymu. Trudy kefedr normalnoi anatomii is histologii s embriologie. Simferopol.

Rudenko, S. (1951): Der zweite Kurgan von Pasyryk im Altai. Berlin.

Rykov, P. (1925): Suslovskij kurgannyj mogilnik. Utsheniie Zapiski Sarat. gos., Univ., Saratov, II, 28; 102.

Rykov, P. (1928): Archäologische Ausgrabungen und Arbeiten an der unteren Wolga im Jahre 1928. Zhurnal Nizhne-Volzhskogo Inst. kraev. im. M. Gorkogo (Saratov).

Rykov, P. (1929): Otshet od arkheol. rabota proizv. v. Nizniem Povolzie letom 1929. Zhurnal Nizhne-Volzhskogo Inst. kraev. im. M. Gorkogo (Saratov).

Rykov, P. (1936): Elista. Izvestiia Saratovskogo Nizhne-Volzhskogo Instituta, VII, 69.

Rzehak, A. (1918): Die römische Eizenzeit in Mähren. Z. d. deutschen Vereins für die Geschichte Mährens und Schlesiens (Brno), XXII, 197-280.

Safar, F. (1947): The history of Eridu, Sumer (Baghdad), III, No. 2, 95-111.

Safar, F. (1949): A preliminary report on the third Season's excavations 1948-1949. Sumer (Baghdad), VI, 27-38.

Salin, E. (1952): La civilization mérovingienne.

Salnikov, K. (1950): Pershino (in Russian). Kratkie Soobshcheniia Instituta Istorii Materialnoi Kulturi, XXXIV, 121.

Salnikov, K. (1953): The Cemetery at Kalmyckii Brod (in Russian). Materialy i issledovaniia po arkheologii SSSR (Moskva), XXXV, 328.

Sauter, M. (1939): Quelques cas de la déformation crânienne arteficielle de l'époque barbare dans la region de Genève. Archives Suisses d'Anthropologie Générale (Genève), 355-360.

Sauter, M. (1945): Les races brachykephales du Proche-Orient des origines a nos jours. Archives Suisses d'Anthropologie Générale (Genève), XI, 68-131.

Sauter, M. (1954-55): Sur des crânes déformés de la nécropole de Saint-Prex, Vaud (VIe siècle). Bull. Soc. Suisse d'Anthropologie et d'Ethnologie, VI-VII.

Schaffhausen, H. (1879): Neue prähistorische Forschungen im Rheinlände. Corr. Bl. dtsch. Ges. Anthropologolie, Ethnologie und Urgeschichte, 124-130.

Schlaginhaufen, O. (1944): Über frühhistorische Gräberschädel aus Mesocco. Bulletin der Schweizerischen Gesellschaft für Anthropologie und Ethnologie, 1943, 8-12.

Schliz, A. (1905): Künstlich deformierte Schädel in germanischen Reihengräber. Arch. Anthrop., N.F., (Braunschweig), Bd. III, 191-214.

Schmidt, B. (1956): Neue Reihengräberfeld im Saalgebiet. Ausgrabungen und Funde, I (Berlin), 228-230.

Schmidt, B. (1961): Künstlich deformierte Schädel und Schädeltrepanationen. Die späte Völkerwanderungszeit in Mitteldeutschland. Veröffentlichungen des Landesmuseums für Vorgeschichte in Halle, Heft XVIII, 160-164.

Schmidt, B., Schott, L. and Schröder, G. (1961): Ein Frauengrab der späten Völkerwanderungszeit mit künstlich deformierten Schädel von Sittichenbach, Kr. Querfurt. Jhschr. f. mitteldt. Vorgeschichte, XLV, 245-251.

Schott, L. (1961): Deformierte Schädel aus der Merowingerzeit Deutschlands in anthropologischer Sicht. In: Schmidt, B.: Die späte Völkerwanderungszeit in Mitteldeutschland. Veröffentlichungen des Landesmuseums für Vorgeschichte in Halle, Heft XVIII, 209-236.

Schránil, J. (1930): Germanské pohrebiste v Zaluzi u Celákovic. Rocenka Okresni jednoty mijezní Brandýs nad Labem, 29-31.

Schránil, J. (1932): Ceskoslovensko v praveku. Csl. Vlastiveda, II. Praha.

Schultz, W. (1941): Die Broschen von Freienbessingen, Kr. Langensalza. Mitteldt. Volkheilk, Bd. VIII (Burg), 16-24.

Schwerz, F. (1915): Die Völkerschaften des Schweiz. Eine anthropologische Untersuchung (Stuttgart), 164.

Senyürek, M. (1955): A note on the long bones of the chalcolithic age from Seyh Höyük. Belleten, XIX, 247-270.

Senyürek, M. and Tunakan, S. (1951): The skeletons of Seyh Höyük. Türk Tarih Kürümü, Belleten (Ankara), XV, No. 60, 438-445.

Sergi, G. (1890): Sopra un cranio deformato. Atti della R. Accademia medica di Roma, XVI, II Ser. (Roma), 16.

Sergi, G. (1908): Description of some skulls from the North Kurgan, Anau (Pumpelly). Explorations in Turkestan. Prehistoric civilization of Anau. Washington.

Sergi, G. (1909-1910): I rilievi cerebrali delle fosse temporale nei crani deformati del Peru. Atti della Societá Romana di Antropologia (Roma), XV, 271-284.

Sinicyn, I. (1936): The Cemetery of Engels-Pokrovsk (in Russian). Izvestiia Saratovskogo Nizhne-Volzhskogo Instituta, VII, 71-81.

Sinicyn, I. (1946): K materialam po sarmatskoi kulture na territorii Niznego Povolzia. Sovietskaia Arkheologia, VIII, 73-95.

Sittenberger, A. (1936): Ein extrem deformierter Schädel aus einem Fürstengrab auf dem Ostgotenfriedhof in Taganrog, Krim. Sitzungsber. Anthrop. Ges., Wien.

Skerlj, B. (1953): Srednjevska okostja z Bleda Izkopana leta 1949. Razprave, Ljubljana.

Skutil, J. (1931): Moravské prehistorické vykopy a nálézy 1930. Sbornik Prirodovedecke spolecnosti v. Mor. Ostrave, VI, 117-171.

Slabe, M. (1970-1971): Grobisce iz dobe preseljevanja narodov v Drevljah. Arheoloski Vestnik (Ljubljana), XXI-XXII, 141-150.

Smirnov, K. (1936): The Cemetery at Tshernokleevsk (in Russian). Arch. Issledovania v. RSFR, 82; Kratkie Soobshcheniia Instituta Istorii Materialnoi Kulturi, XXXIV, 107.

Smirnov, K. (1948): Sarmatskie progrebenia iuzhnava Priuralia. Kratkie Soobshcheniia Instituta Istorii Materialnoi Kulturi (Moskva-Leningrad), XXII, 80ff.

Smirnov, K. (1953): The Cemetery at Ilovatki (Volgograd) (in Russian). Sovietskaia Arkheologia, XVIII, 138.

Smirnov, M. (1877): Sur les fouilles enterprises dans la région du Caucase. Bulletin de la Societe d'Anthropologie de Paris, 3me Serie, I, 541-553.

Snorzason, E. (1946): Cranial deformation in the region of Akhnaton. Bull. History of Medicine, XX, No. 5, 601-610.

Steinburg, M. (1874): Ein Schädelfund von Székelyudvarhely u. Mitteilung über einige andere Schädel. Hermannstadt, 1874, 1875. Prog. d. Evang. Gymnasiums in Schässburg, 1-36.

Stloukal, M. (1965): Künstlich deformierte Schädel von Vyskov. Anthrop. Anzeiger XXIX. Festband Gieseler (Stuttgart), 250-260.

Sturms, E. (1953): Das Problem des ethnischen Deutung der kaiserlich zeitliche Gräberfelder in der Ukraine. Zeitschrift für Ostforschung, II, 425ff.

Straub, A. (1881): La cimetière Gallo-Romain de Strassbourg. Strassburg.

Svoboda, B. (1939): Böhmen in der Völkerwanderungszeit. Acta Musei Nationalis Pragae I, 157-200.

Svoboda, B. (1965): Cechyv dobe stehovaní narodu. Praha.

Szepura ? (1875): Versuch einer anthropologischen Erforschung der makrokephalen Schädel, die in der Grüften des alten Kirchhofs von Somtour gefunden wurden. Tiflis (in Russian).

Tanakan, S. (1951): The skeletons from Seyh Höyük. Belleten, XV, 439-445.

Thaeringen, G. (1939): Die Nordharzgruppe der Elbgermanen bis zur sächsischen Überlangerung. Berlin.

Thompson, D'Arcy, W. (1941): On Growth and form.

Topinard, P. (1879): Des déformations ethniques du crâne. Bulletin de la Société d'Anthropologie de Paris, 2me série, II, 496-506.

Török, A. (1884): A koponya mesterséges eltozításáról. Ttud. Közl., XVI, 225ff.

Török, A. (1884): Makrocephale Schädel und Anderes. Correspondenzblatt d. Anthrop. Ges. (München), XV, 177-179.

Török, A. (1887): A koponya mesterseges eltorzításáról. (Uber die künstliche Schädeldeformation). Ttud. Közl., XIX, 261-265.

Török, A. (1903): Bericht über die macrocephalen Schädel aus Velem. Mitteilungen der Anthrop. Ges. in Wien, XXXIV, 35-48.

Török, A. (1904): Uber einen neueren Fund von makrokephalen Schädeln aus Ungarn. Ztschr. Morph. Anthrop., VII, 141-201.

Török, A. (1907): Az emberi koponya mesterseges eltorzításáról és tüzetesebben a makrokephalokról. (Über die künsliche Deformierung des menschlichen Schädels und genauer über die Makrokephalen.) Magy. Orv. és Term. vizsg., (Vándorgyűlése), XXXV, 223-226.

Török, A. (1907): A koponya mesterséges eltorzításáról és a magyarországi kaukázusi makrocephalokról. (Uber die Schädeldeformierung und die Makrokephalen aus Ungarn und dem Kaukazus.) Ttud. Közl., XXXIX, 603ff.

Török, Gy. (1935): A kiszombori germán temető helye népvándorláskori emlékeink között. Szeged. Szeged városi nyomda és könyvkiadó, 56.

Trapp, M. (1872): Die Heidengräber nächst des Bahnhofes bei Znaim. Mitt. der kais. königl. Mährisch-Schläsischen Ges. für Ackerbau- und Landkunde (Brno), LII, 392-400.

Trofimova, T. (1941): Schädel aus dem Gräberfeld von Lugovoj. Arbeiten aus dem Anthropologischen Institut, VI (in Russian).

Trofimova, T. (1959): Drevnee naselenie Horezma po dannym paleoantropologii (Moskva), 102.

Trofimova, T. (1961): Paläoanthropologie des Mittelasiens. Anthropogiai Közlemenyek (Budapest), V, 1-4, 69-87.

Trofimova, T. and Ginzburg, V. (1960): Antropologitsheskii sostav naselenia juznoi turkmenii v epohu eneolita. Trudy juznoturkmenskoi komplexoi expedicii (Ashabad), X, 478-528.

Troyon, F. (1841): Description des tombeaux de Bel-Air, près Chessaux-sur-Lausanne (Lausanne), Mitt. der antiquarischen Ges. in Zürich

Troyon, F. (1864): Classification des crânes humaines dans ma collection d'antiquites. IN: Rütimeyer, L. and His, W.: Crania Helvetica (Basel), 1-58.

Troyon, F. (1965): On the Crania Helvetica. Annual reports of the Board of Regents of the Smithsonian Institution, 282-284.

Tschudi, J. (1845): Ein Awarenschädel. Archiv für Anatomie und Physiologie, 277-280.

Turnovszky, J. (1879): A human artificially deformed skull found in Hungary. New York Odontological Society, 168-171.

Ujfalvy, C. (1898): Memoire sur les Huns blances (Hephtalites de l'Asie centrale, Huns de l'Inde) et sur la deformation de leurs crânes. Anthropologie (Paris), IX, 395ff.

Ullrich, H. (1957): Trois crânes artificiellement déformés du Bas-Rhin. Bulletin de la Société d'Anthropologie de Paris, VIII, 10me série, 276-283.

Uvarova, P. (1902): Sammlungen des Kaukas (in Russian) (Tbilisi), V, 159.

Vallois, H. (1937): Notes sur les ossements humains de la Nécropole énéolitique de Byblos. Bull. du Musée de Beyrouth, I, 23-33.

Vallois, H. (1939): Les ossements humains de Sialk. In: Girsham, R.: Fouilles de Sialk 1933, 1934, 1937, Vol. II, 113-192.

Verneaux, R. (1927): A propos de la déformation du crane chez les Mambouttous de l'Quelle. Bull. Musée d'Hist. Naturelle, IV, 1-8.

Veselovskij, N. (1902): Kurgany Kubanskoi oblasti v period rimsk. cladicestva na Severnom Kavkaze, Trudy XII. Arch. S'ezda Kharkov, 341ff.

Virchow, R. (1873): Bericht über die vierte Versammlung der Deutschen Gesellschaft für Anthropologie, Ethnologie und Urgeschichte zu Wiesbaden im Jahre 1870. Zeitschrift für Ethnologie (Berlin).

Virchow, R. (1888): Das Gräberfeld von Osorukova (Urushbevo). Zeitschrift für Ethnographie, XX, 406ff.

Virchow, R. (1890): Excursion nach Lengyel. Verhandlungen der Berliner Gesellschaft für Anthropologie, Ethnologie und Urgeschichte (Berlin), XXII, 97-118.

Virchow, R. (1891): Schädel und Skeletteile aus Hügelgräber der Hallstatt und La Tene Zeit in der Oberpfalz. Verhandlungen der Berliner Gesellschaft für Anthropologie, Ethnologie und Urgeschichte (Berlin), 359-365.

Virchow, R. (1896): Defekte des os tympanicum an künstlich deformierten Schädeln von Pomeraniern. Verhandlungen der Berliner Gesellschaft für Ethnographie, 69-74.

Virchow, R. (1901): Über Schädelform und Schädeldeformation. Korr. Bl. Dt. Ges. für Anthropologie, XXXIII, 135-139.

Virchow, R. (1902): Besuch der Höhlen von St. Canzian bei Triest. Verhandlungen der Berliner Gesellschaft für Anthropologie, Ethnologie und Urgeschichte (Berlin), 225-231.

Vjasmitina, M. (1953): The Cemetery at Novo-Filipovka (in Russian). Arkheologiia (Kiev), VIII, 62.

Vlcek, E. (1952): Umele deformorovaná lebka z Klucova. Archeologické rozhledy, IV, 112-130.

Vlcek, E. (1957): Umele deformorovaná lebka ze Slovenska. Jansákov sborni, Nitra.

Vlcek, E. (1957): Anthropologicky material z obdobi stehovaní národo na Slovensku. Antropologické pracovisko Archeologického ustavu Slovenská Akademia Vied. Bratislava, V, No. 2, 402-434.

Voisin, A. (1866): Présentation de moules craniens. Bulletin de la Société d'Anthropologie de Paris, 2me Série, I, 99-100.

Vram, U. (1896): Nota sopra un cranio deformato. Atti della Società Romana di Antropologia, (Roma), III, 173-175.

Vram, U. (1897): Ancora sul macrocefalo della grotta Tominz di S. Canziano. Seduta della Società Antropologia del 15 Maggio 1897. Roma.

Vram, U. (1898): Sopra un caso di macrocefalia ippocratica. Atti della Società Romana di Antropologia (Roma), fasc. 1, 89-92.

Waldeyer, W. (1881): Types des Têtes. In: Straub, A.: Le cimetière gallo-romain de Strassborug. Strassbourg.

Weisbach, E. (1875): Erenköl. Mitt. d. Anthrop. Ges. in Wien, V, 153-157 and XII, (1882), 77-80.

Weissenberg, S. (1927): Ein Fall von Turmschädel. Anthrop. Anzeiger (Stuttgart), IV, 44-46.

Werner, J. (1956): Beiträge zur Archäologie des Attila-Reiches. Bayerische Akademie der Wissenschaften. Philosophisch-historische Klasse. Abhandlungen. N.F. Heft XXXVIII A. München.

Werner, J. (1958): Neue Daten zur Verbreitung der artifiziellen Schädeldeformation im I. Jahrtausend n. Ch. Germania, XXXVI, 162-164.

Wilson, D. (1862): Ethnical forms and undesigned distortions of the human cranium. Toronto.

Zakharov, A. (1930): The Cemetery at Tyemir-Chan-Shura, Eurasia (in Russian). Septentrionalis Antiqua, V, 183ff.

Ziegel, K. (1939): Die Thüringe der späten Völkerwanderungszeit im Gebiet östlich der Saale. Jehresschrift für die Vorgeschichte der sächsisch-thüringischen Länder, XXXI. Abschnitt "Die deformierten Schädel" (Halle), 64-66.

Zirov, E. (1940): Ob iskusstvennoi deformacii golovy. Kratkie Sobstshenia Instituta Istorii Materialnoi Kultura (Moskva-Leningrad), VIII, 81-88.

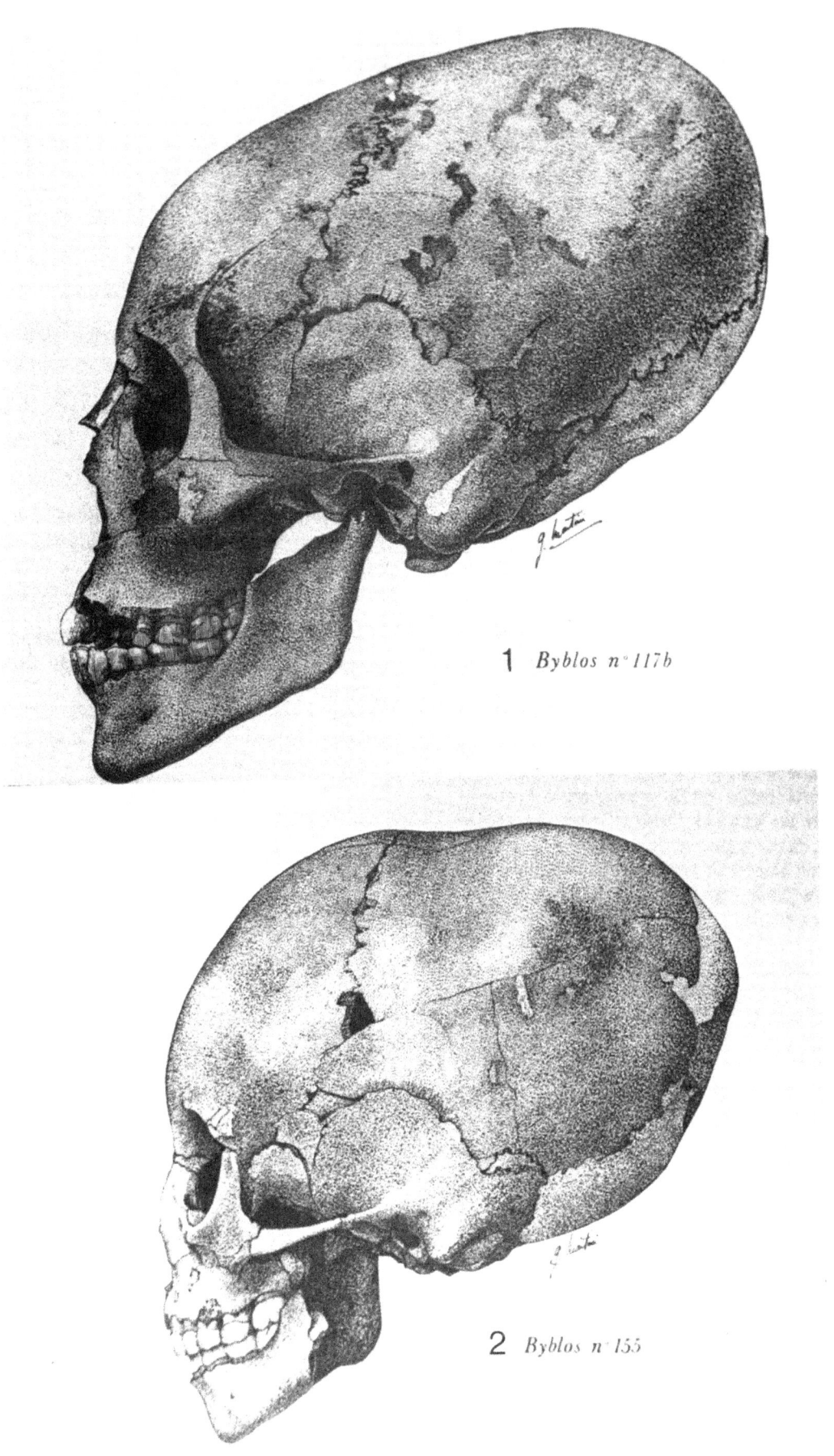

Fig. 1 Artificially formed skulls from Byblos, Lebanon

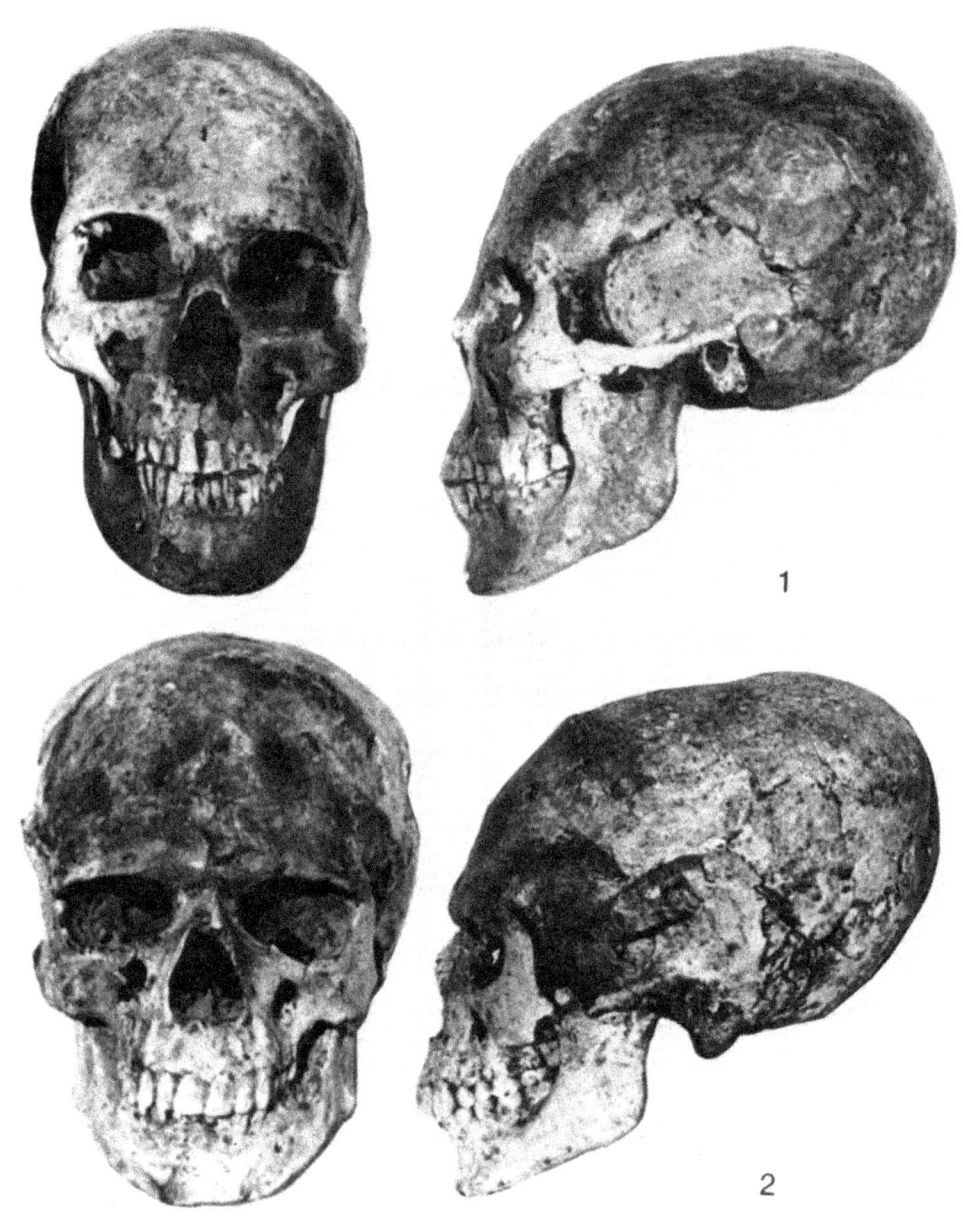

Fig. 2   Artificially formed skulls from Eridu (Tell Abu Shahrain), Iraq.
1. Grave 1; 2. Grave 2.

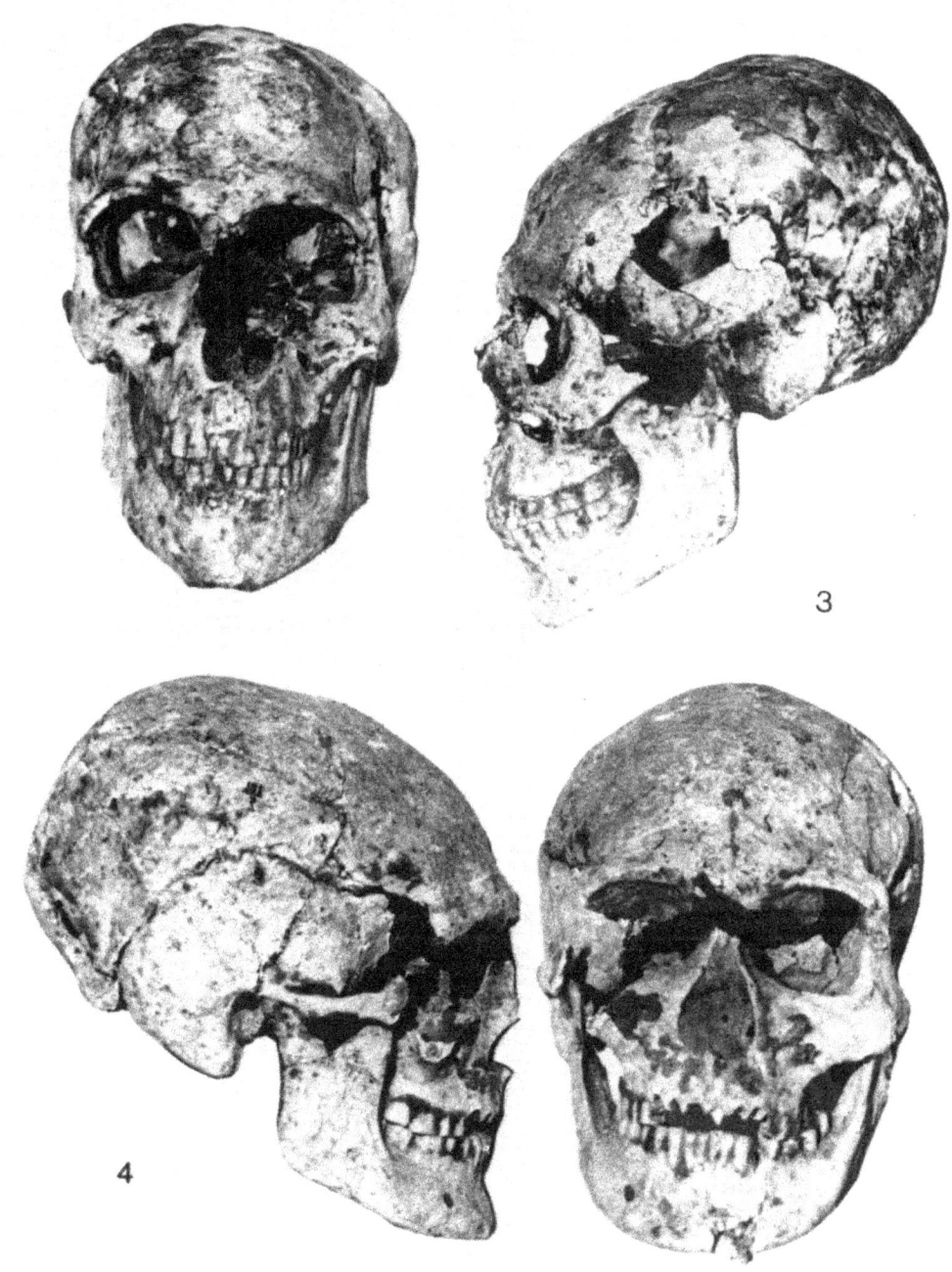

Fig. 3 Artificially formed skulls from Eridu (Tell Abu Shahrain), Iraq.
3. Grave 116; 4. Grave 181.

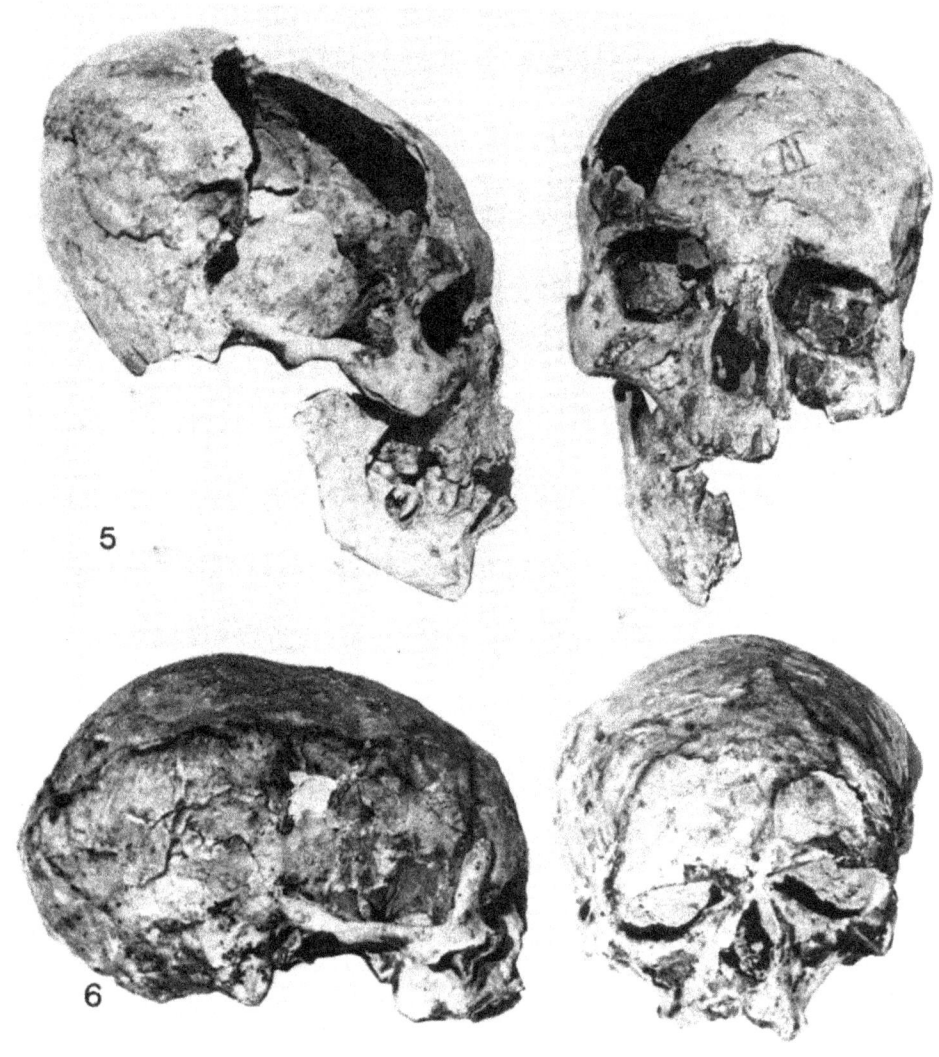

Fig. 4 Artificially formed skulls from Eridu (Tell Abu Shahrain), Iraq.
5. Grave III; 6. Grave X_1.

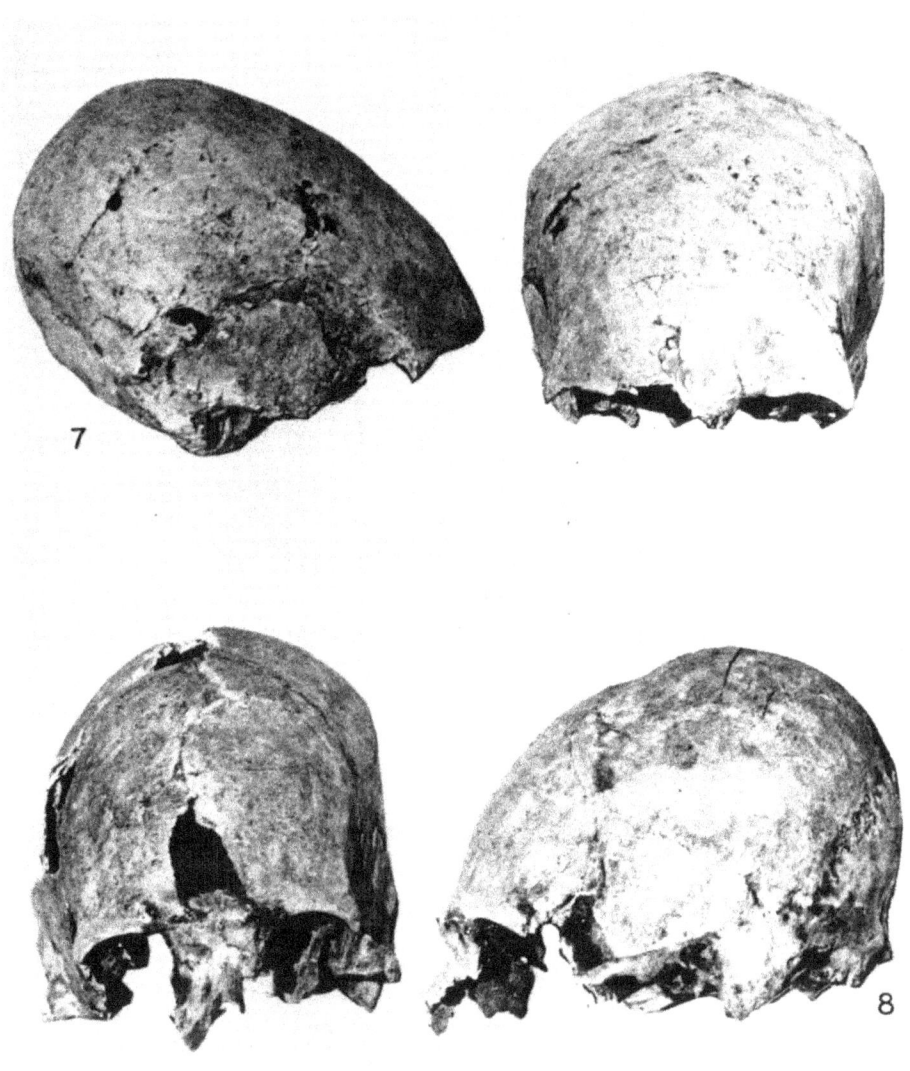

Fig. 5 Artificially formed skulls from Eridu (Tell Abu Shahrain), Iraq. Grave No. IV; 8. Grave X_2.

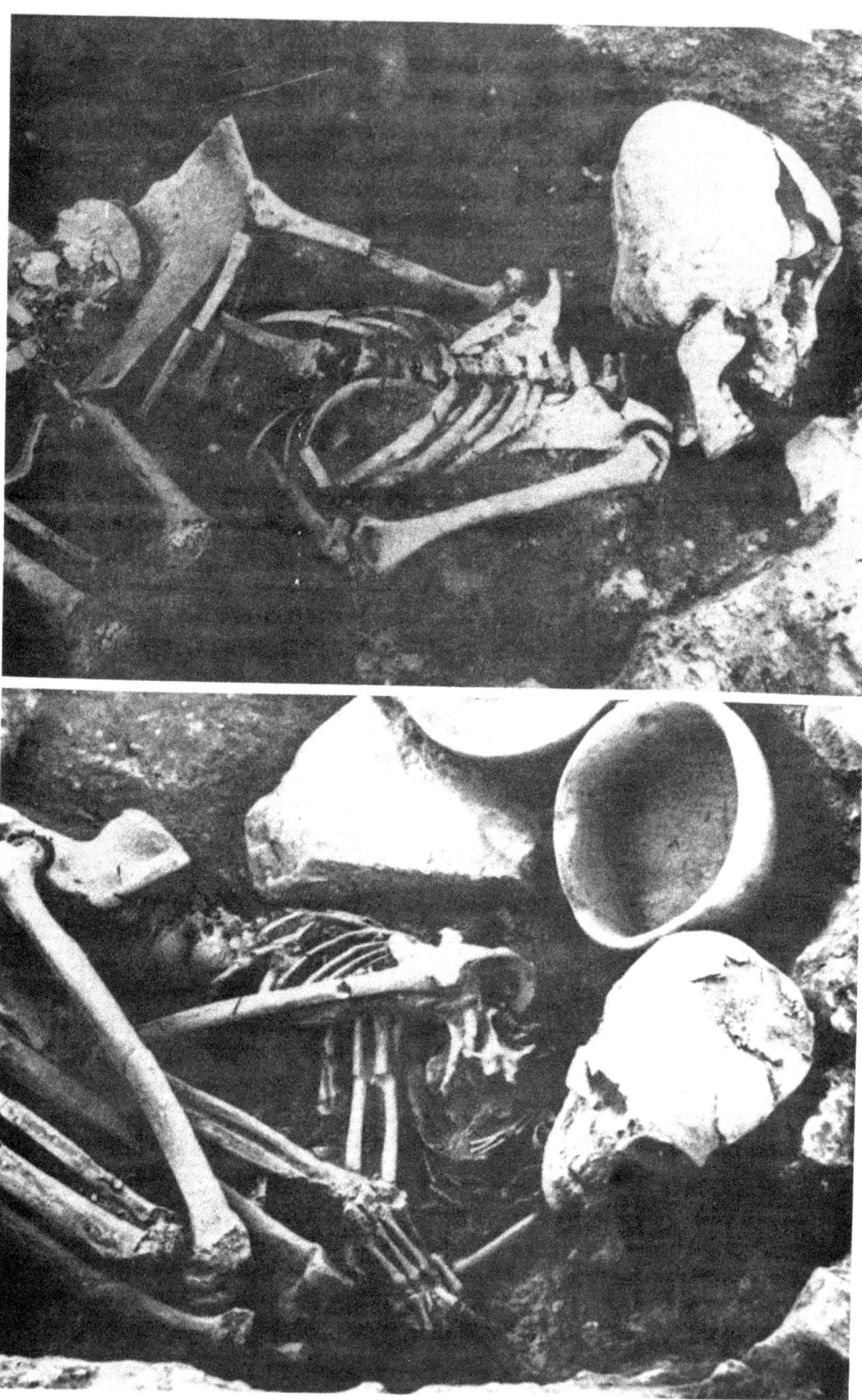

Fig. 6   Artificially formed skull in situ, from the Cemetery at Khirokitia, Cyprus

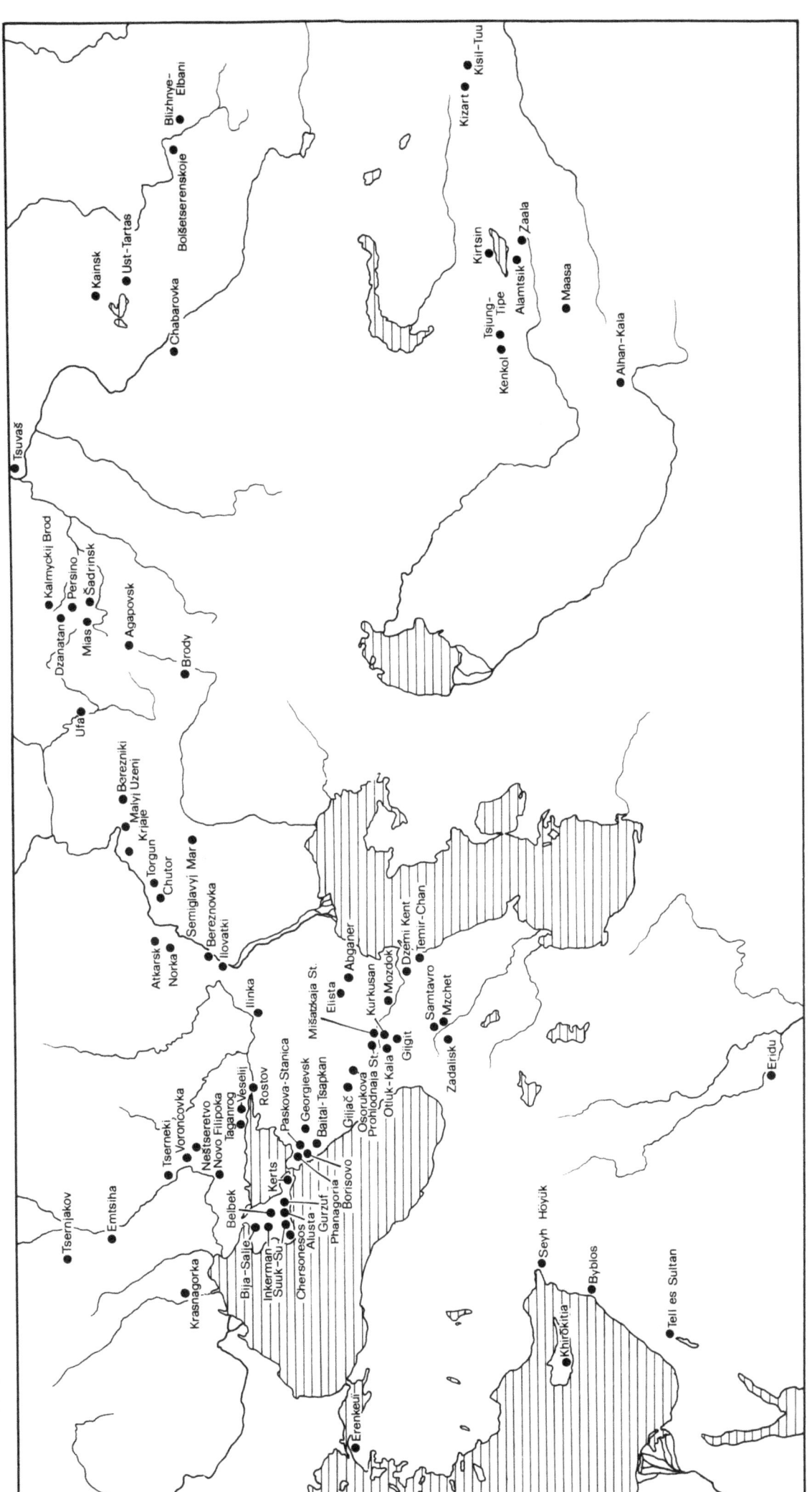

Fig. 7 Sites where artificially formed skulls have been found in the Near East and the Soviet Union.

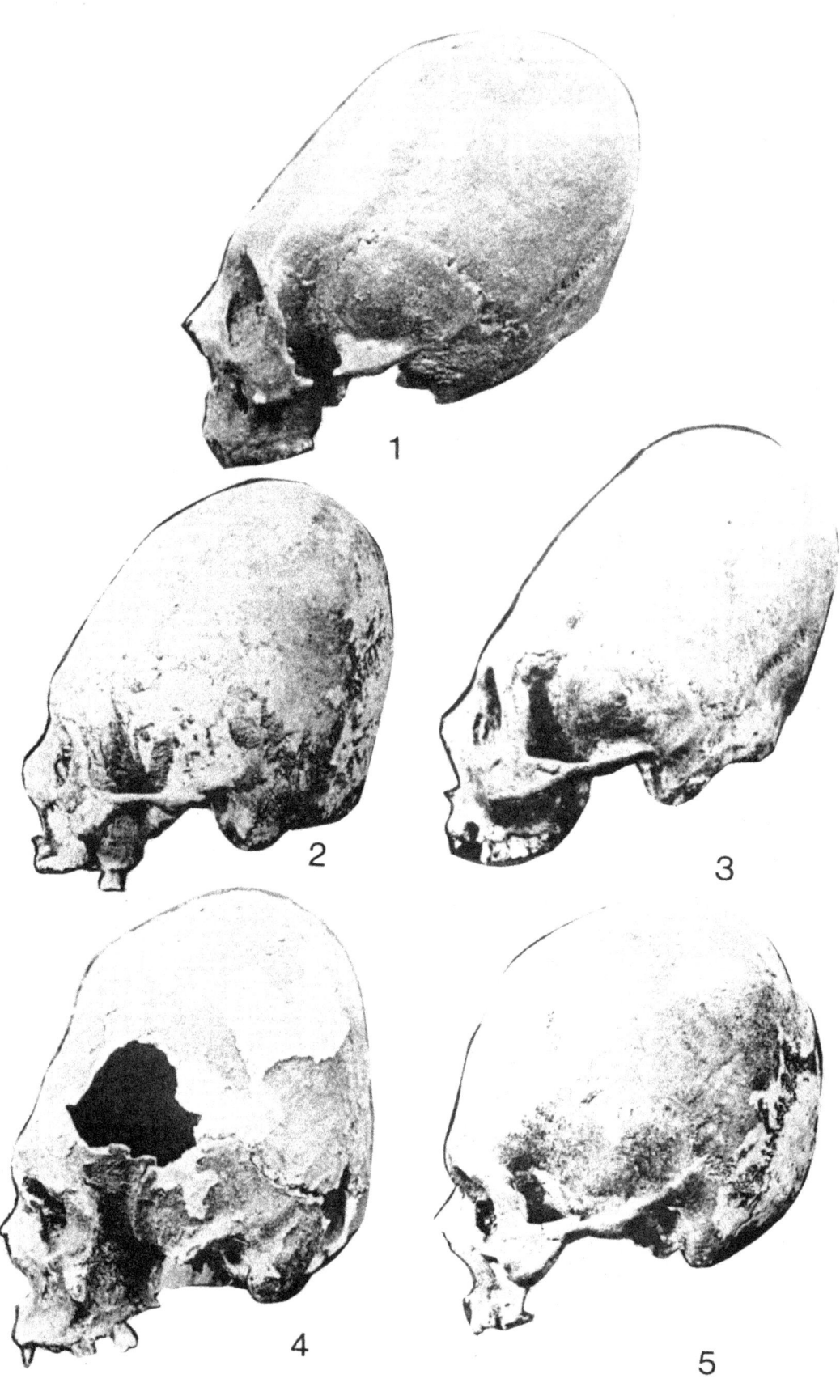

Fig. 8 Artificially formed skulls from Ordzonikidze (Dzaudzhikau), Caucasus

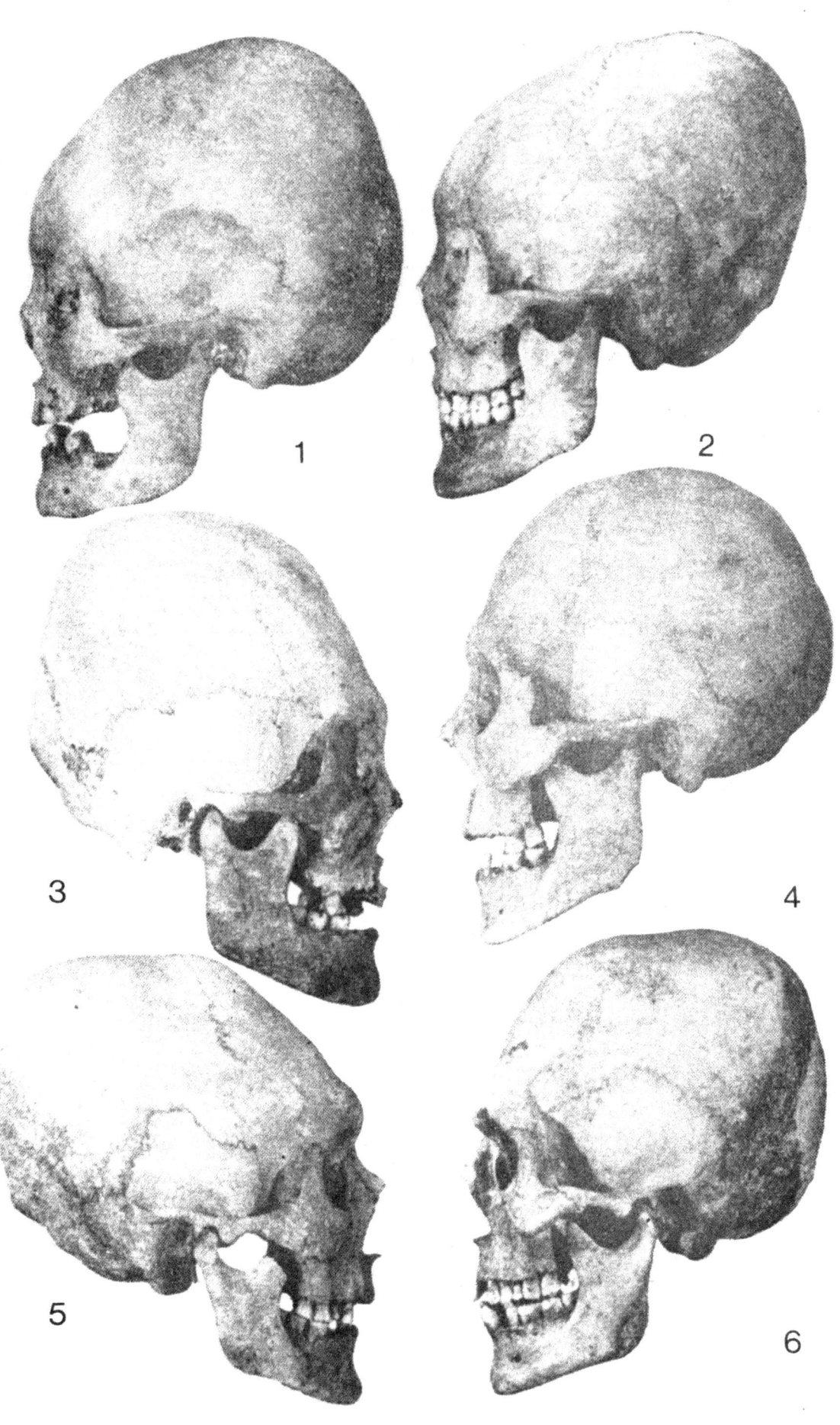

Fig. 9 Artificially formed skulls from the U.S.S.R. 1. Bereznovka, kurgan 59; 2. Bereznovka, kurgan 40; 3. Bereznovka, kurgan 40; 4. Skatovka, kurgan 5; 5. Bereznovka, kurgan II; 6. Rovnij, kurgan 9.

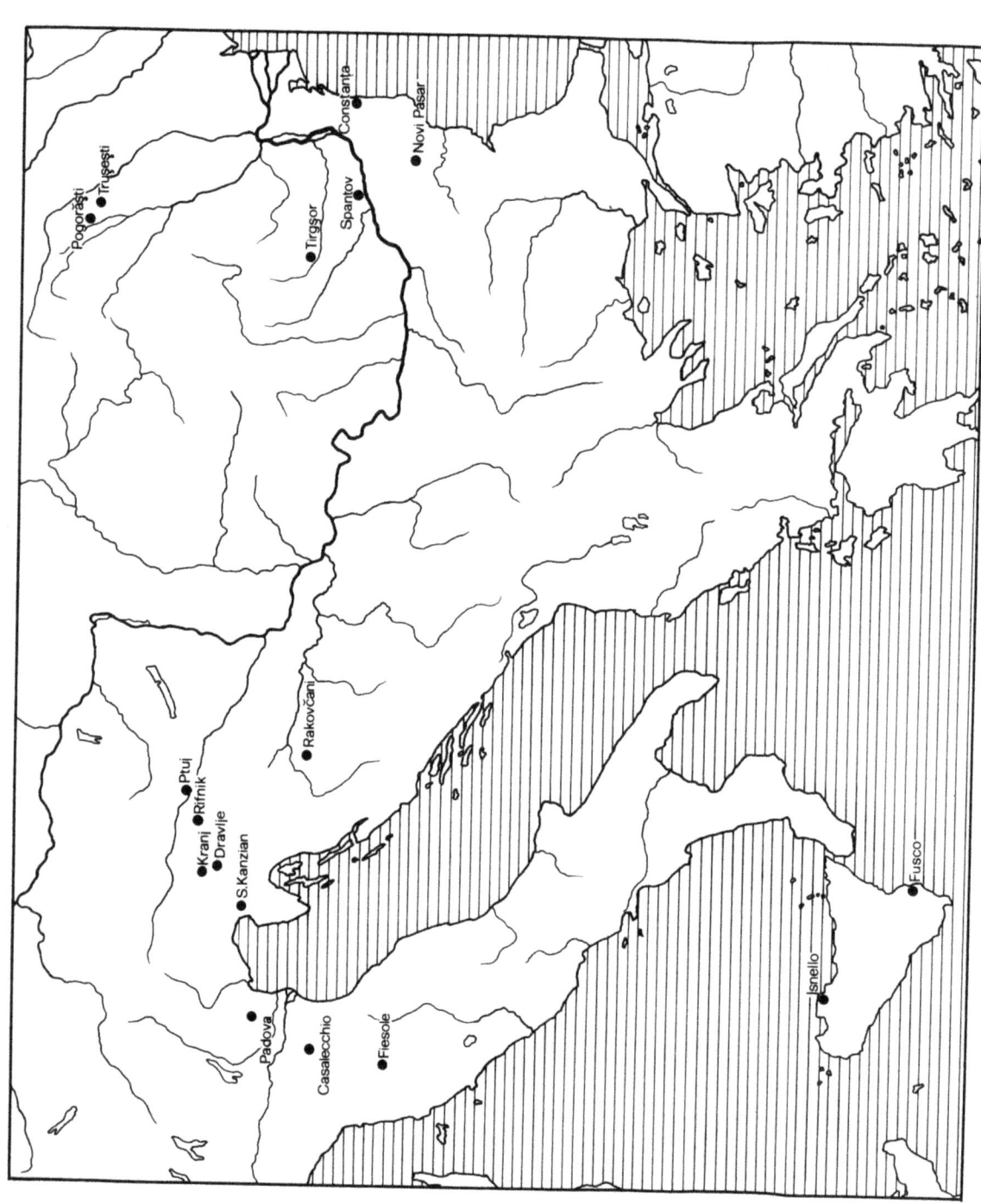

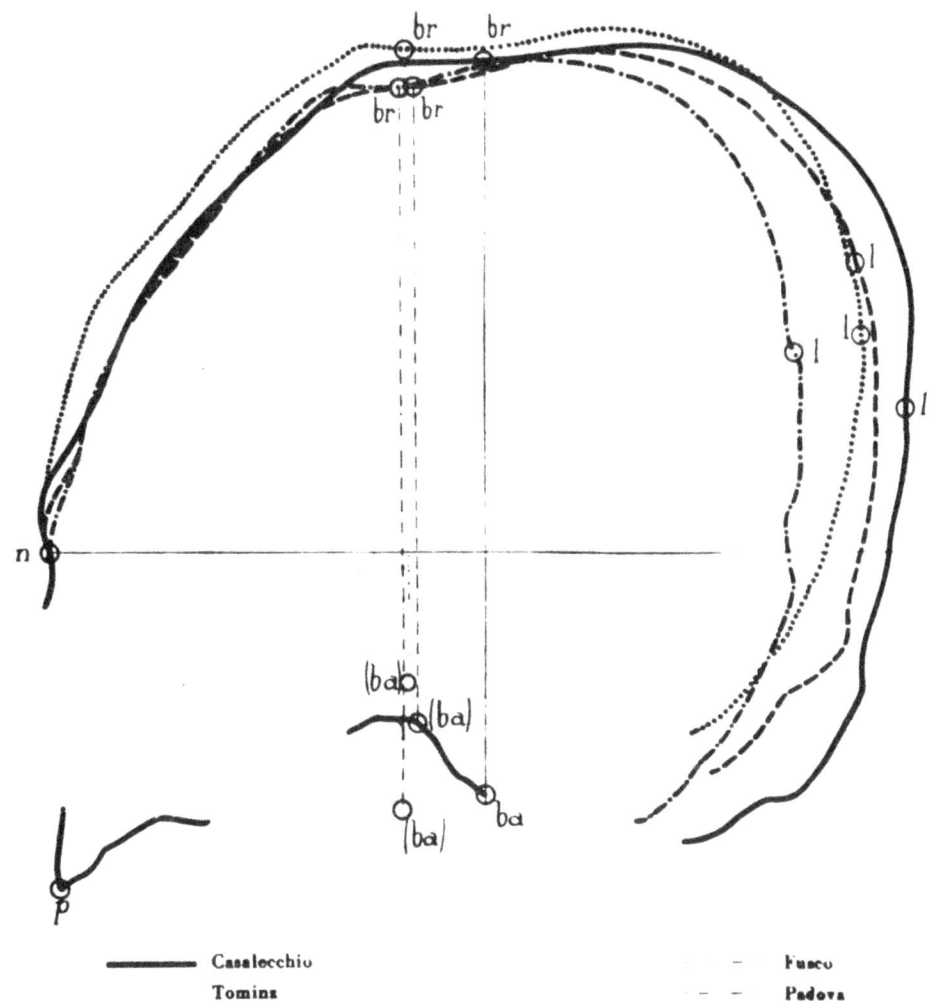

Fig. 11 Differences between some artificially formed skulls found in Italy (<u>Norma</u> <u>lateralis</u>)

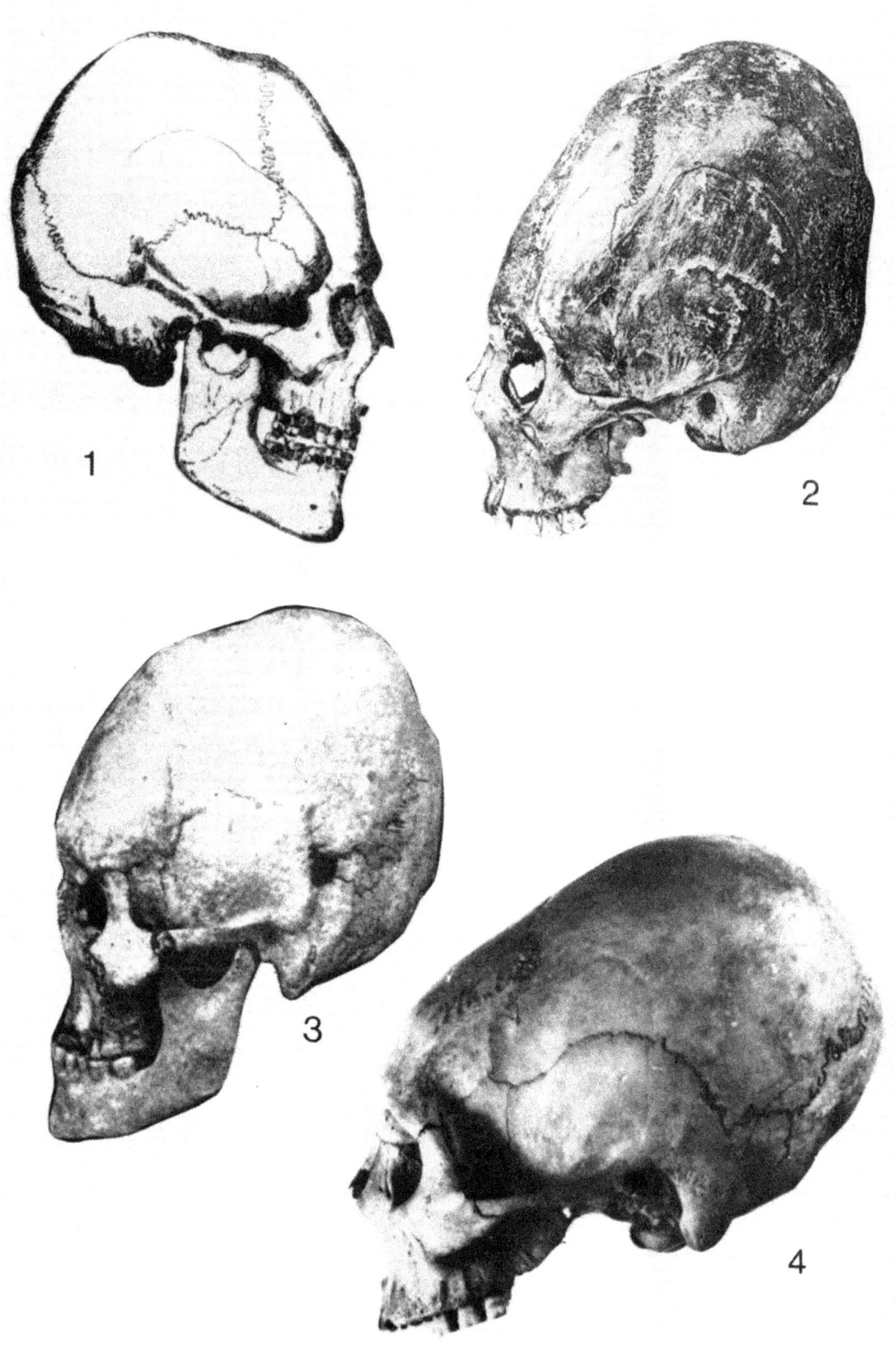

Fig. 12 Artificially formed skulls from Romania, Hungary and Greece.
1. Székelyudvarhely (Romania); 2. Csongrád (Hungary);
3. Pogorásti (Romania); 4. Trikeri (Volos-Thessalia), Greece.
The last was found in the nineteenth century.

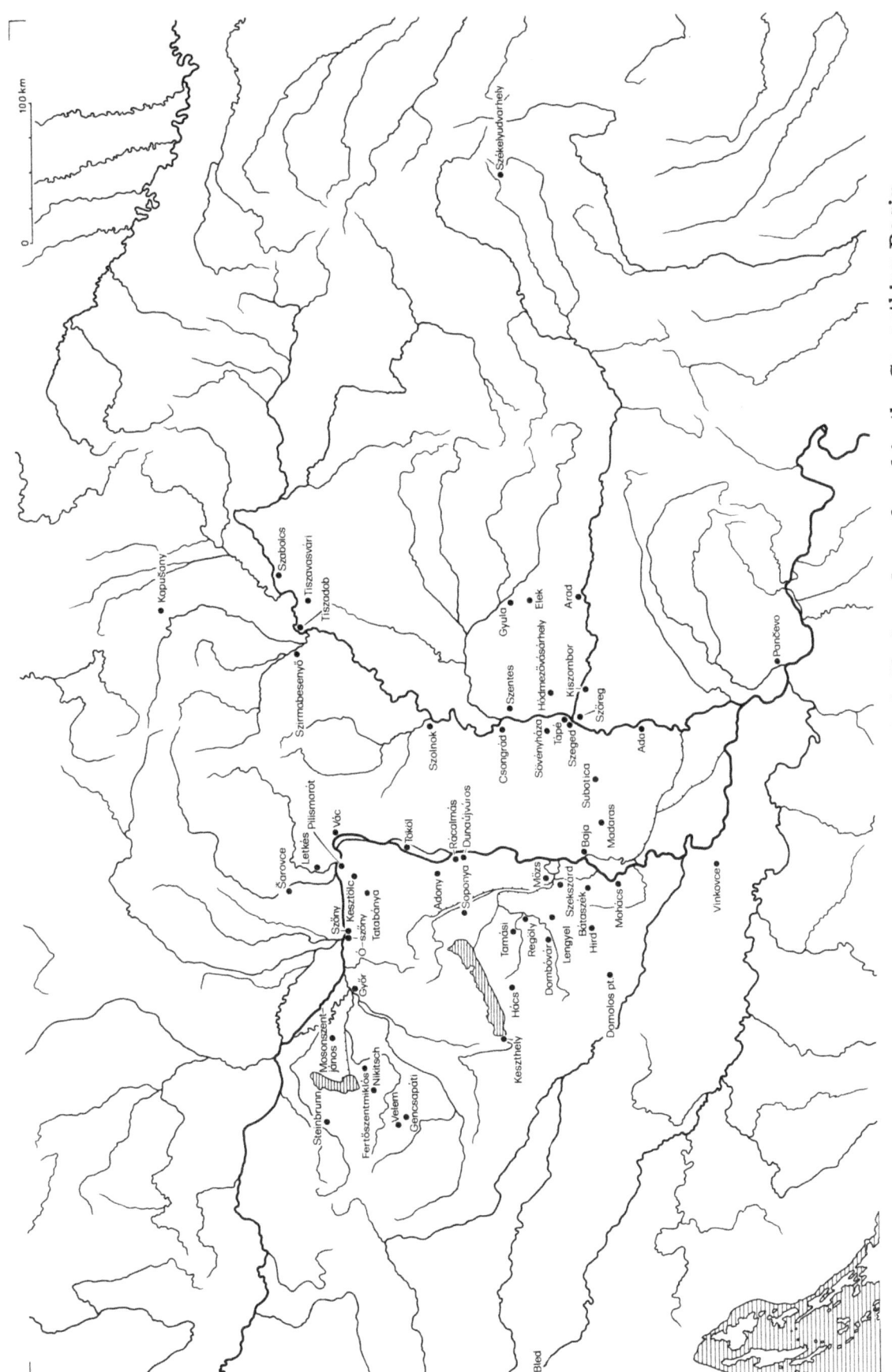

Fig. 13 Sites where artificially formed skulls have been found in the Carpathian Basin.

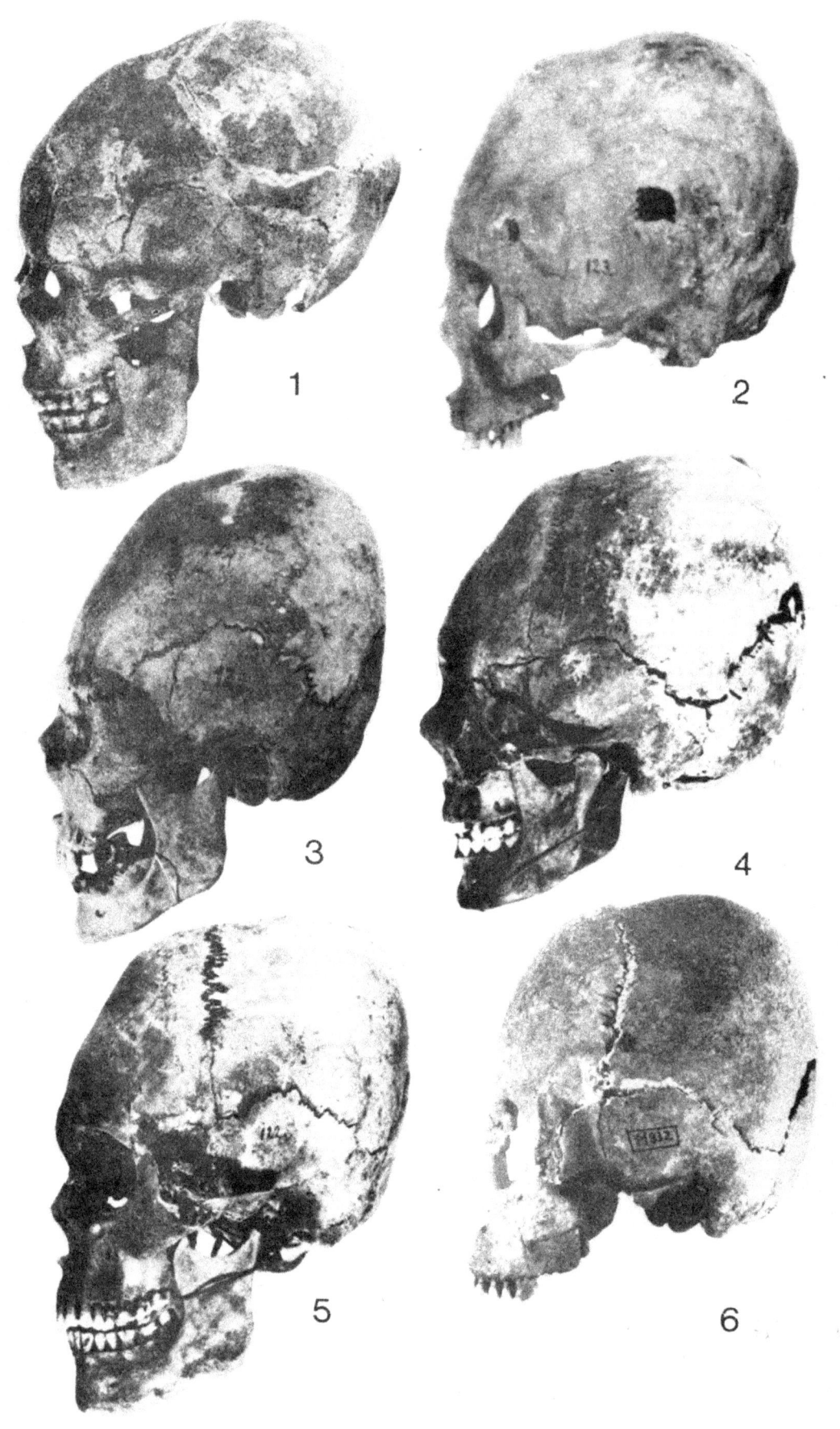

Fig. 14 Artificially formed skulls from Southern Hungary.
1. Kiszombor B, grave 25; 2. Koszombor B, grave 123;
3. Koszombor B, grave 389; 4. Kiszombor B, grave 234;
5. Kiszombor B, grave 43 and Szőreg, grave 85.

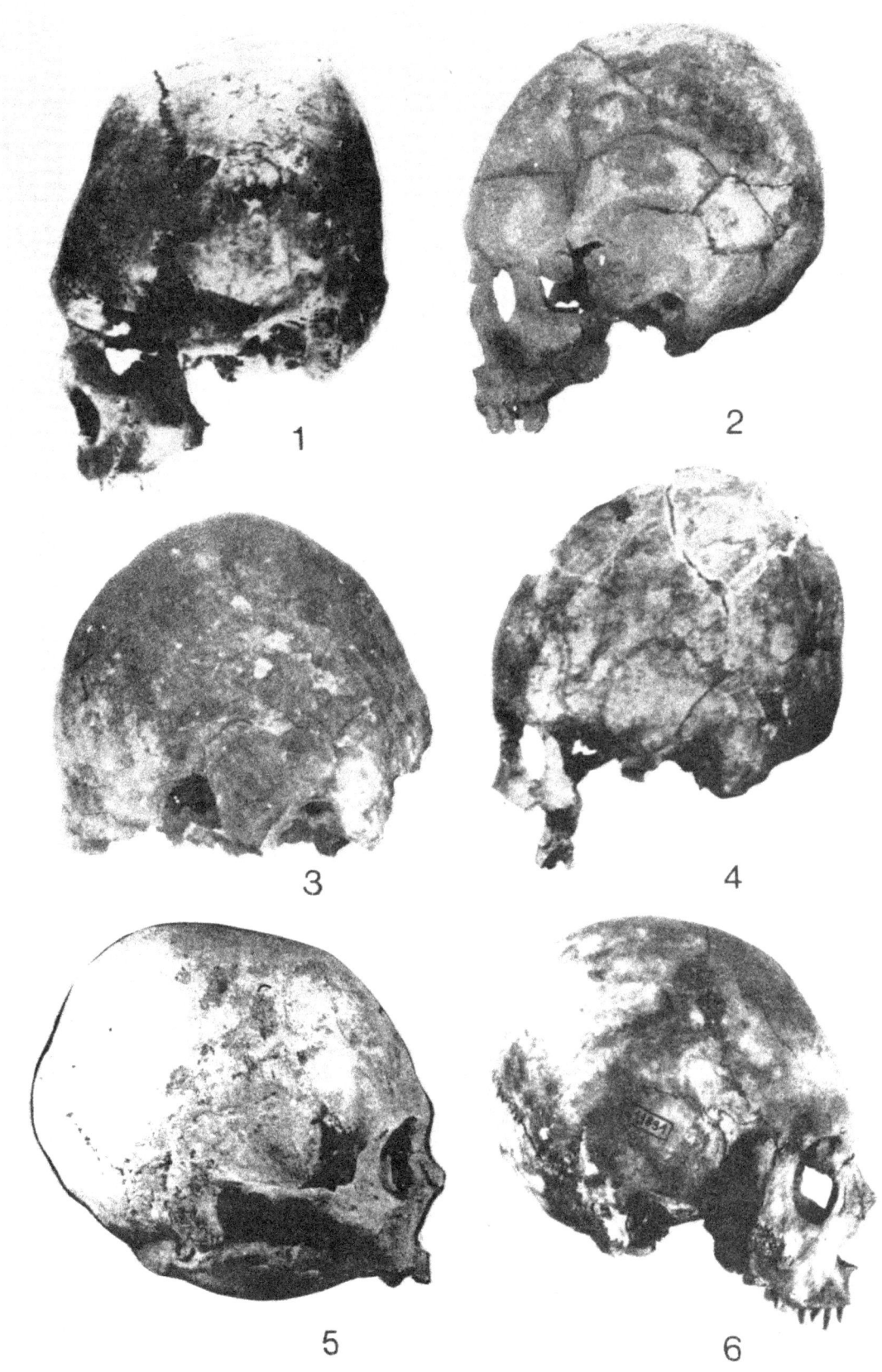

Fig. 15 Artificially formed skulls from Southern Hungary.
1. Szőreg, grave 126; 2. Kiszombor B, grave 109;
3. Kiszombor B, grave 57; 4. Szőreg, grave 89;
5. Kiszombor B, grave 225; 6. Szőreg, grave 75.

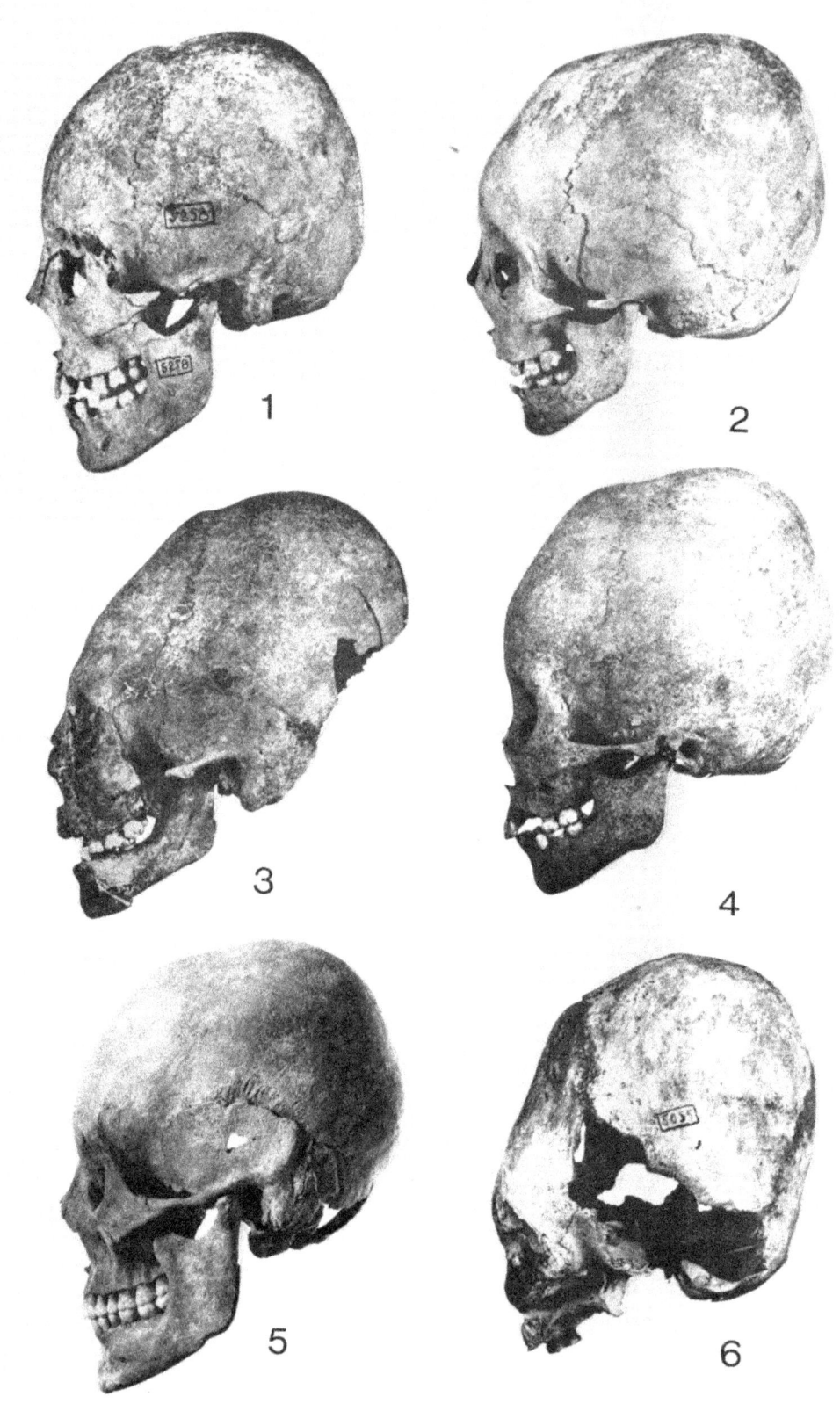

Fig. 16 Artificially formed skulls from Hungary.
1. Mohács; 2. Keszthely-Fenékpuszta; 3. Győr;
4. Győr-Szechenyi-tér; 5. Regöly; 6. Adony.

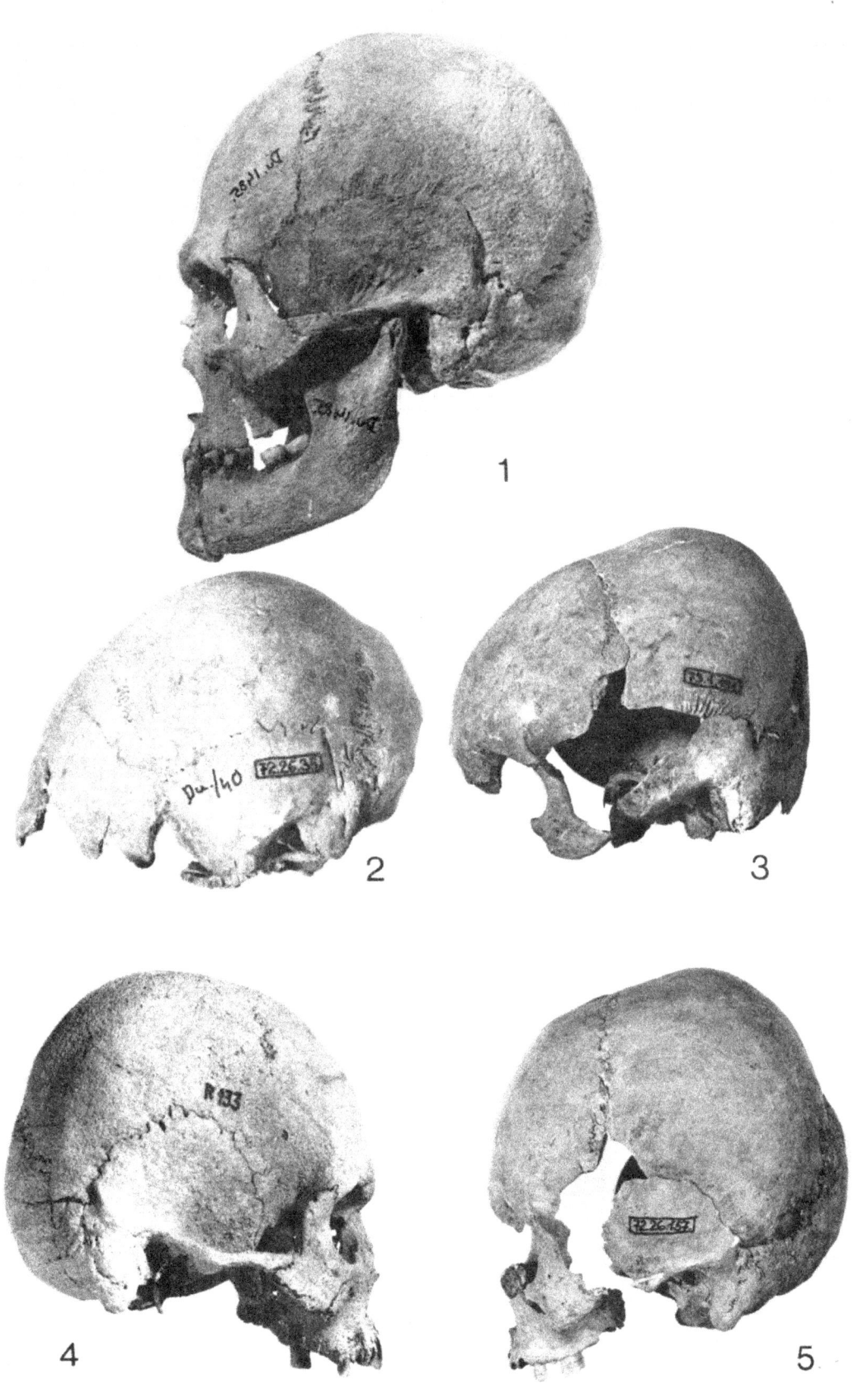

Fig. 17 Artificially formed skulls from Hungary.
1. Intercisa (Dunaujváros), grave 1485; 2. Intercisa, grave 40;
3. Intercisa, grave 600/c; 4. Rácalmás, grave 133; 5. Intercisa, grave 210.

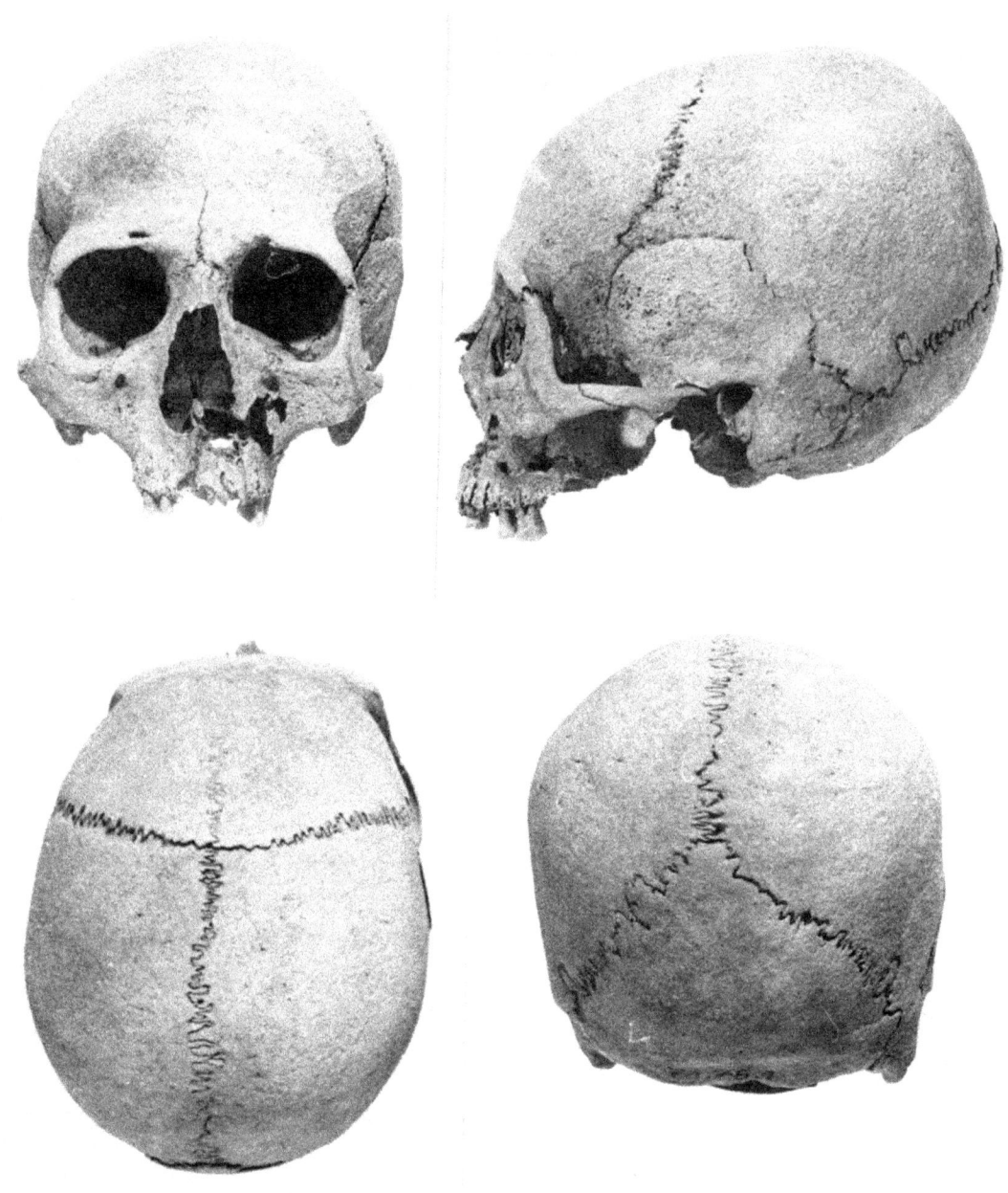

Fig. 18 Artificially formed skull viewed along 4 axes, from Fertőszentmiklós, Hungary.

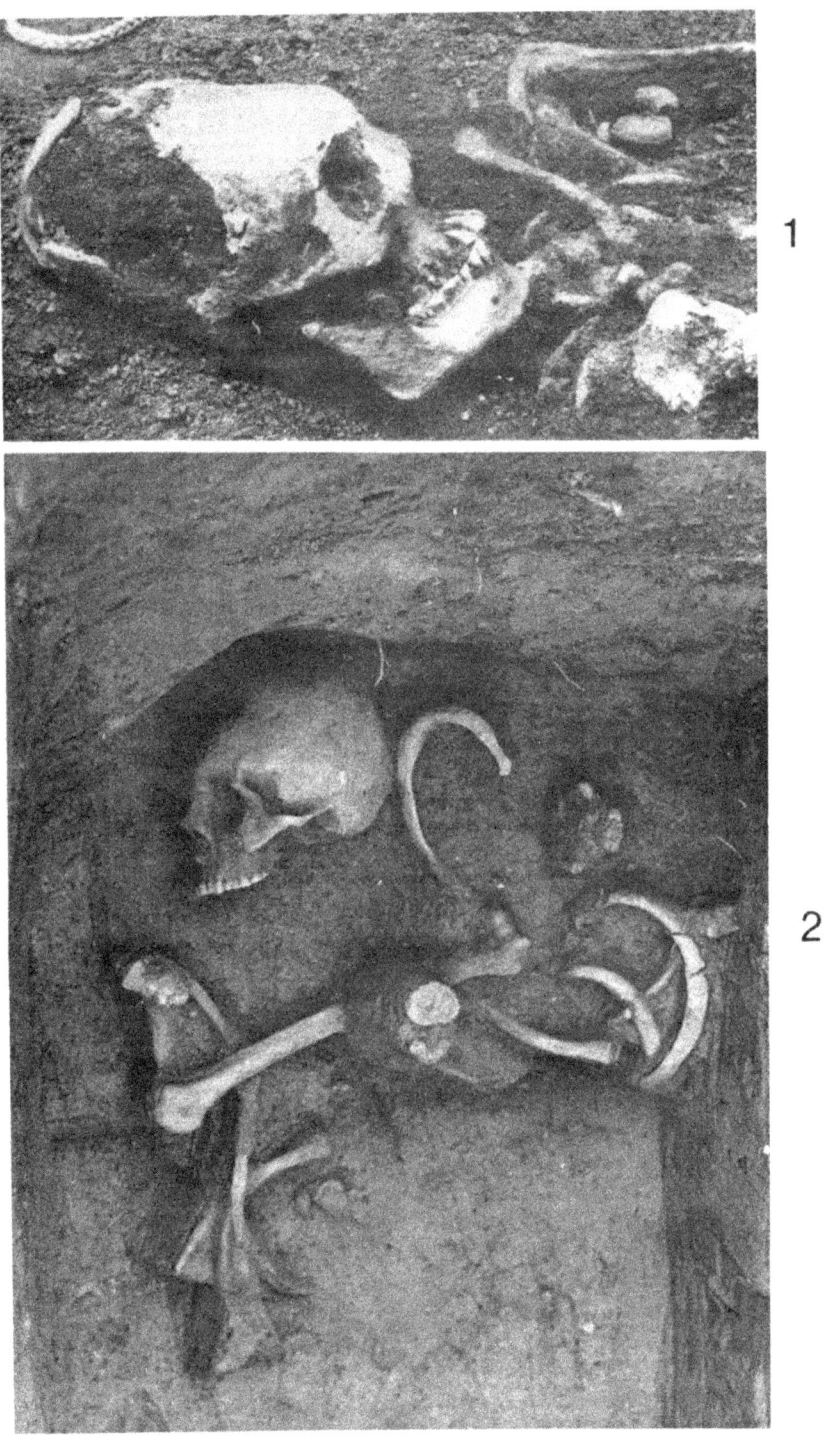

Fig. 19 Artificially formed skulls in situ.
1. Ingersleben; 2. Keszthely-Fenékpuszta.

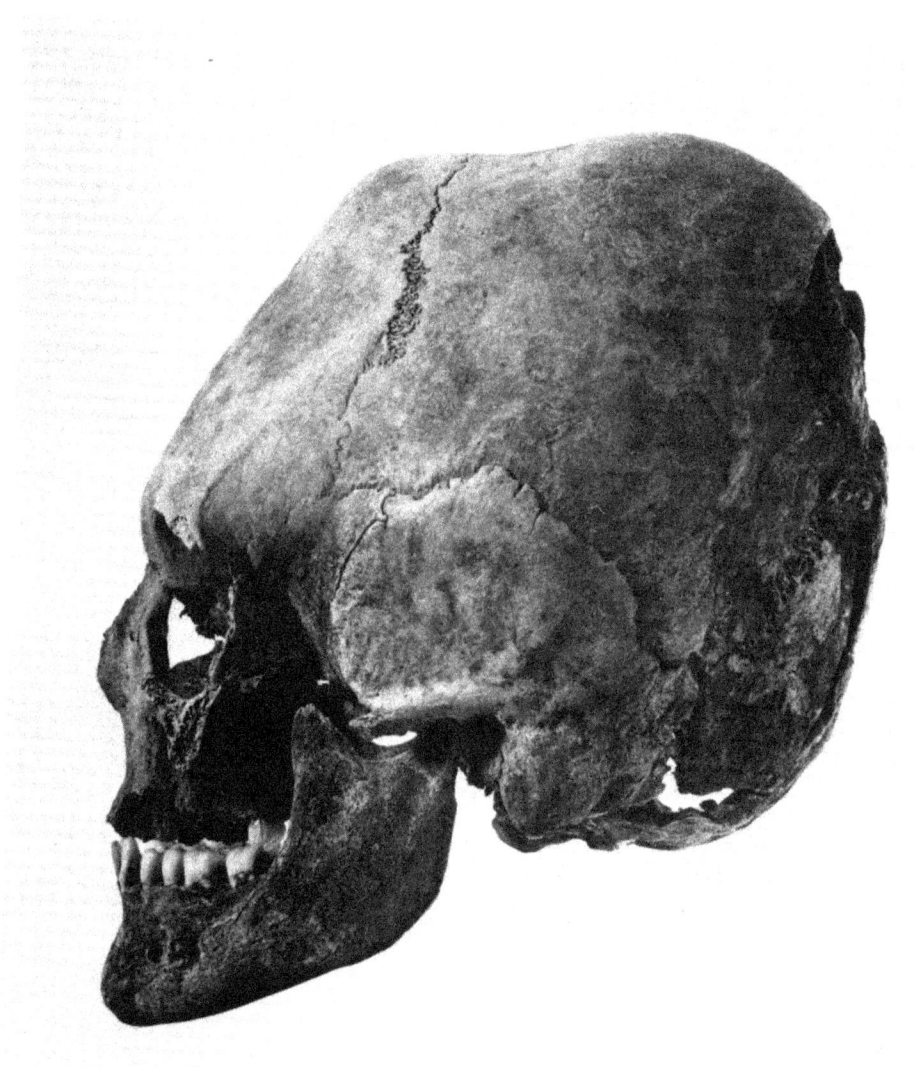

Fig. 20 Artificially formed skull from Soponya (Hungary), Grave 2.

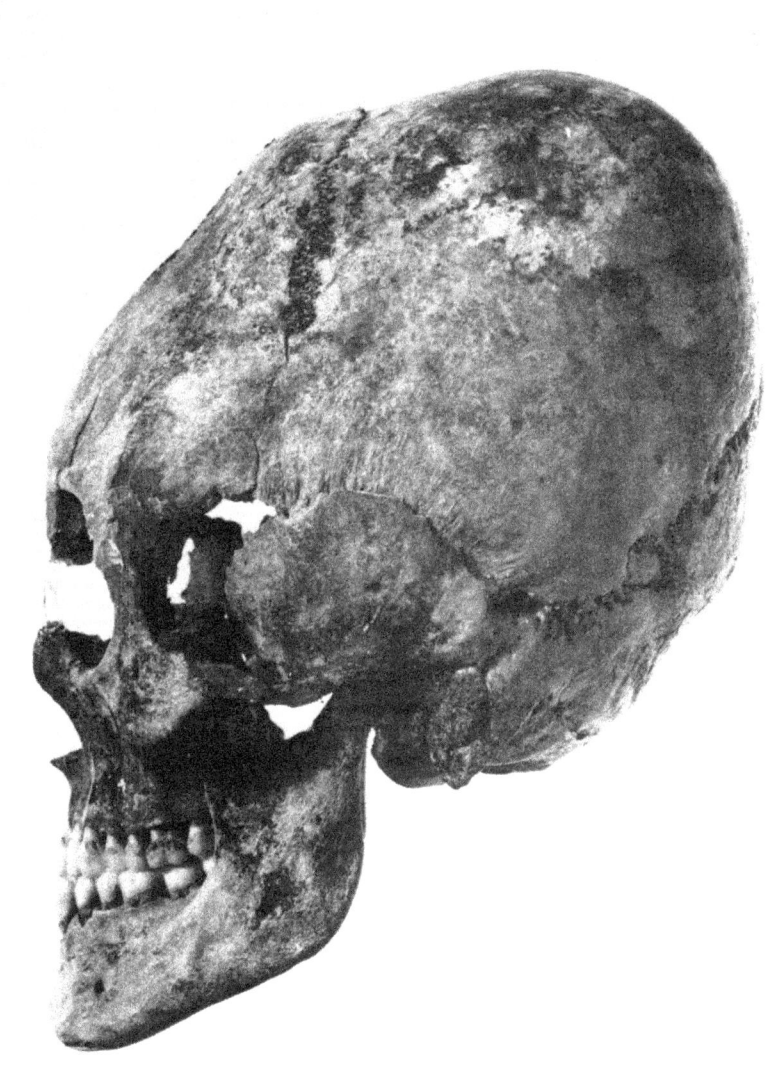

Fig. 21 Artificially formed skull from Soponya (Hungary), Grave 4.

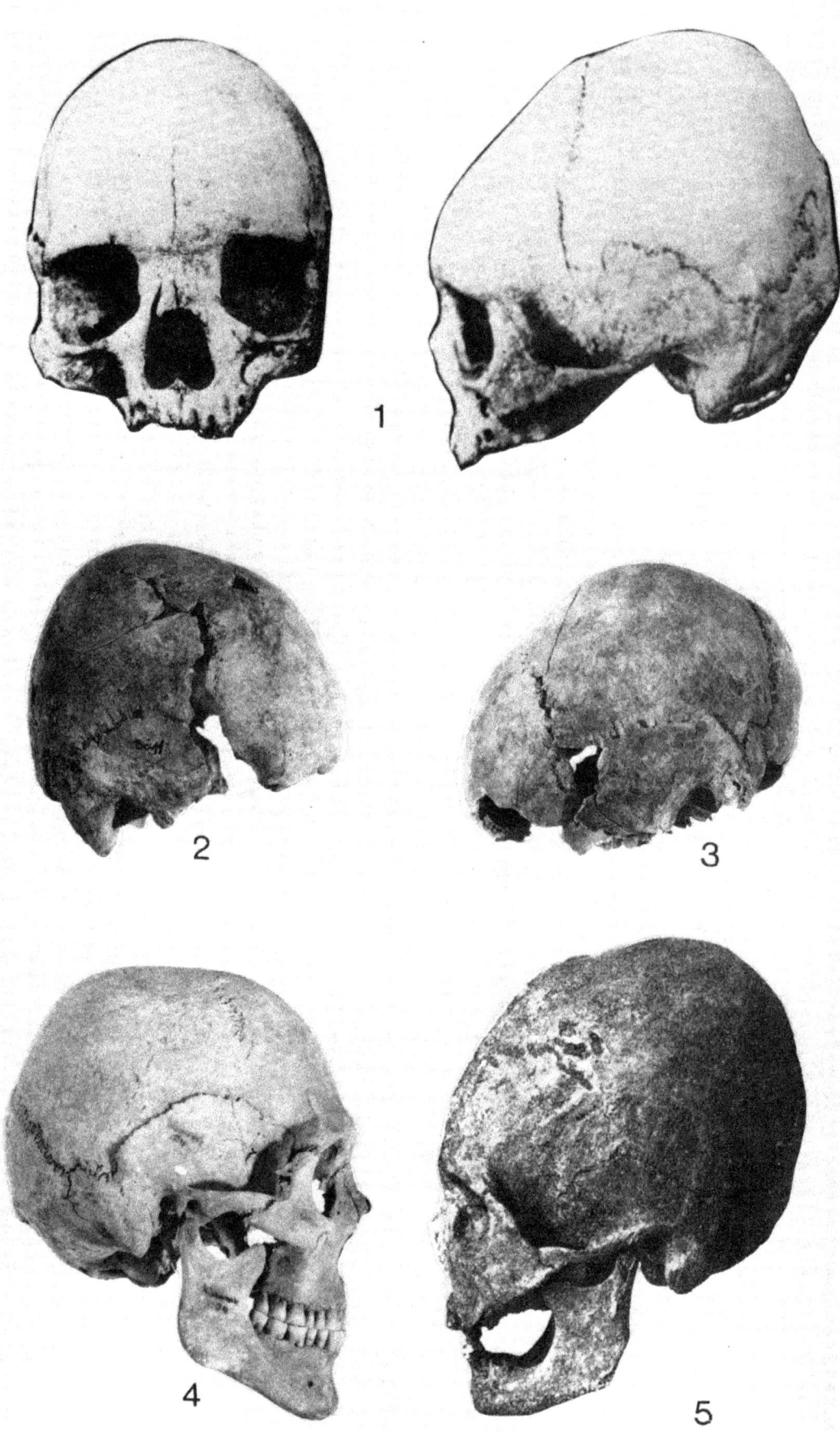

Fig. 22 Artificially formed skulls from Hungary.
1. Tököl; 2. Bökény, grave 11; 3. Bökény, grave 15;
4. Hódmezővásárhely-Kishomok; 5. Hódmezovásárhely-Gorzsa.

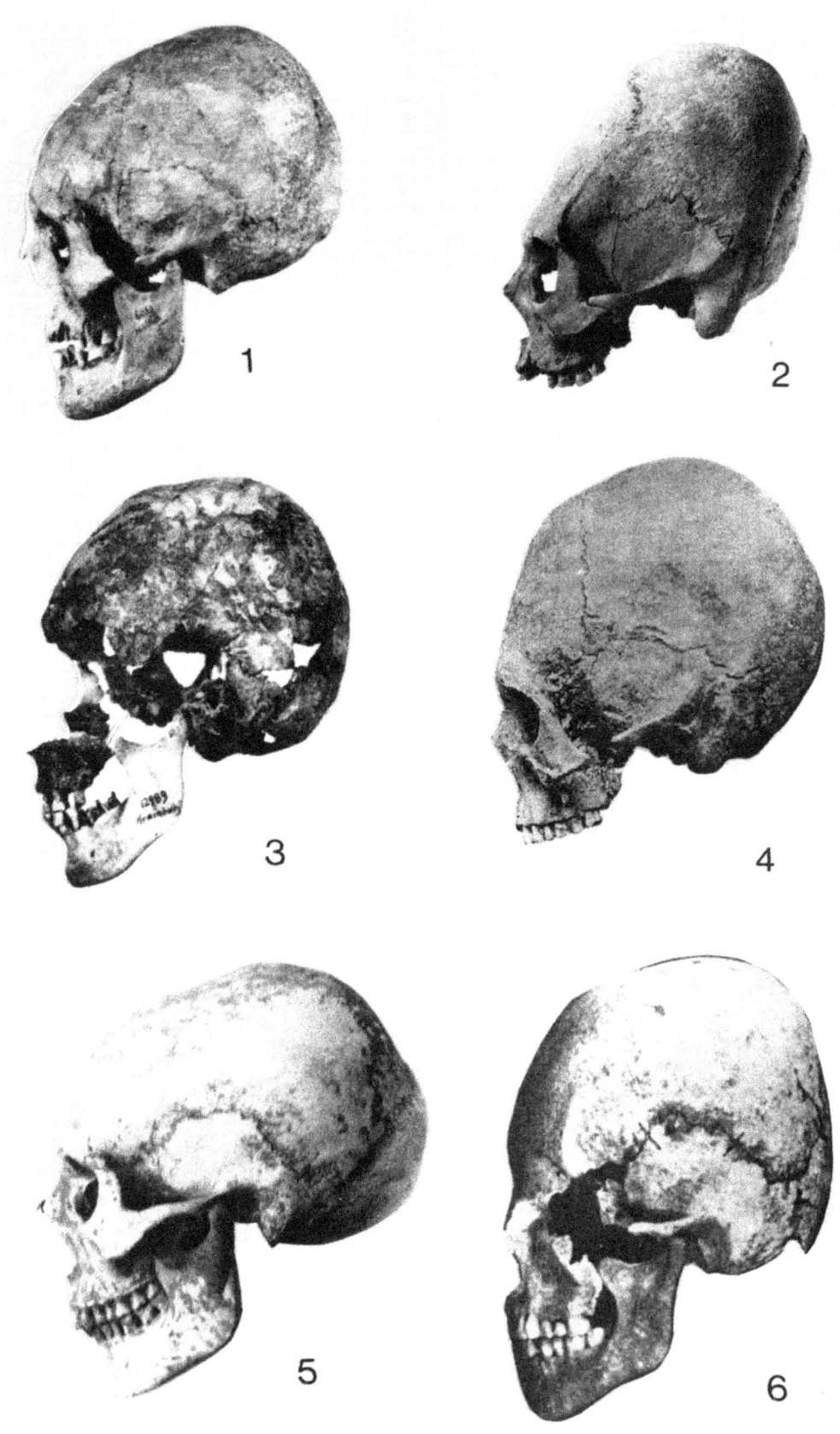

Fig. 23 Artificially formed skulls from Central and Southern Europe.
1. Nikitsch, grave 2 (Austria); 2. Tamási-Adorjánpuszta (Hungary); 3. Kranj (Jugoslavia); 4. Praha-Podbaba (Czechoslovakia); 5. Fiesole (Italy); 6. Novi-Pasar (Bulgaria).

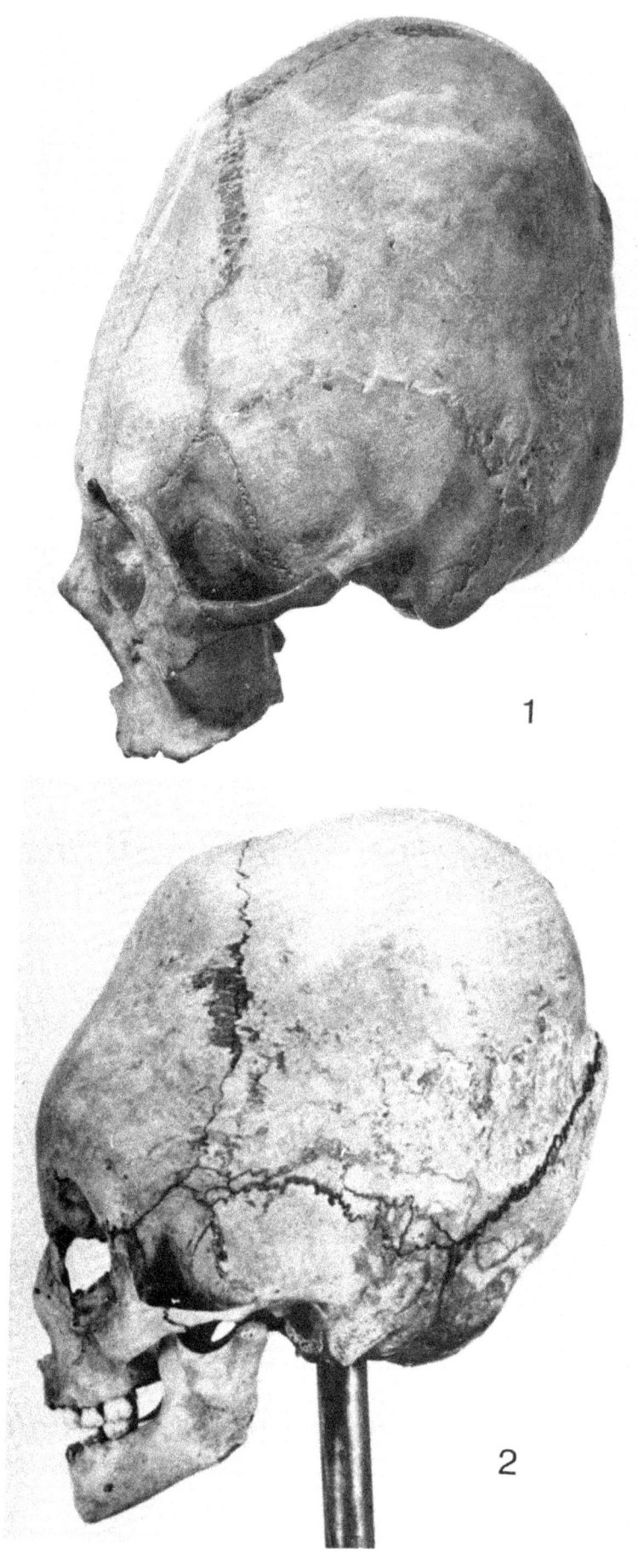

Fig. 24 Artificially formed skulls from Austria.
1. Grafenegg; 2. Burgstall.

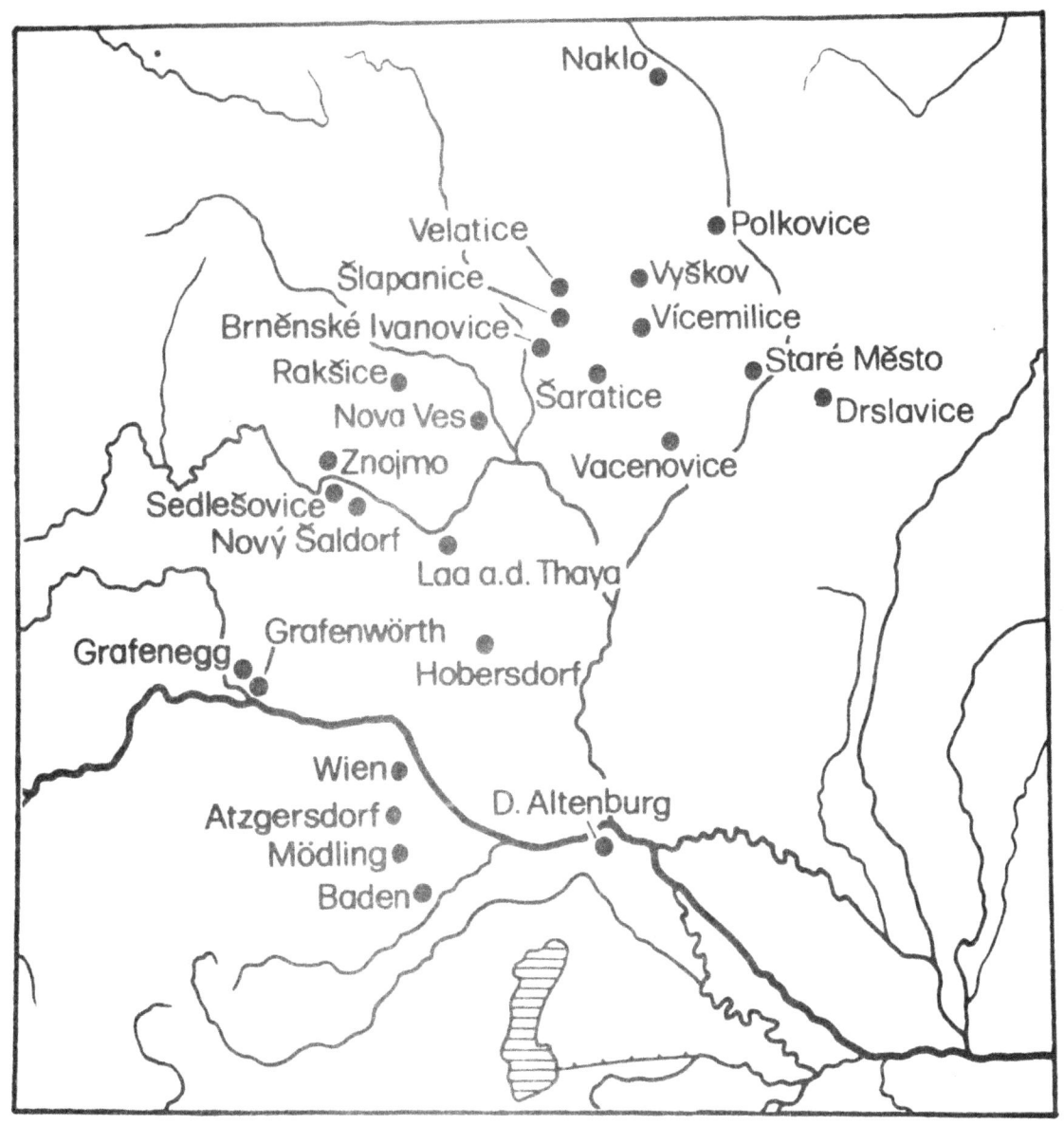

Fig. 25 Sites in the territory of the Rugii and in the Vienna region where artificially formed skulls have been found.

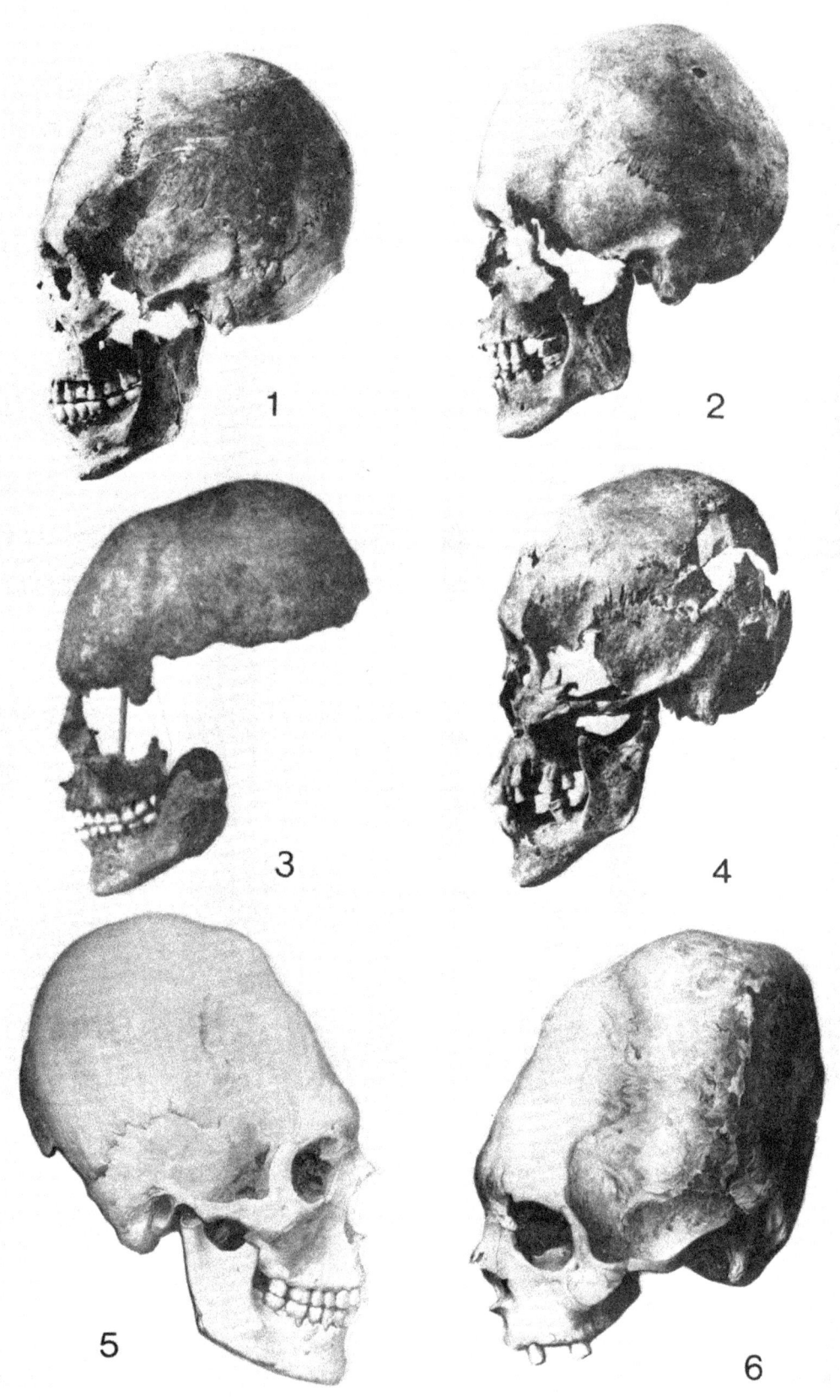

Fig. 26 Artificially formed skulls from Austria.
1. Hobersdorf, grave 3; 2. Wien-Salvatorgasse, grave 21;
3. Hobersdorf; 4. Wien-Salvatorgasse, grave 2;
4. Atzgersdorf; 6. Grafenegg.

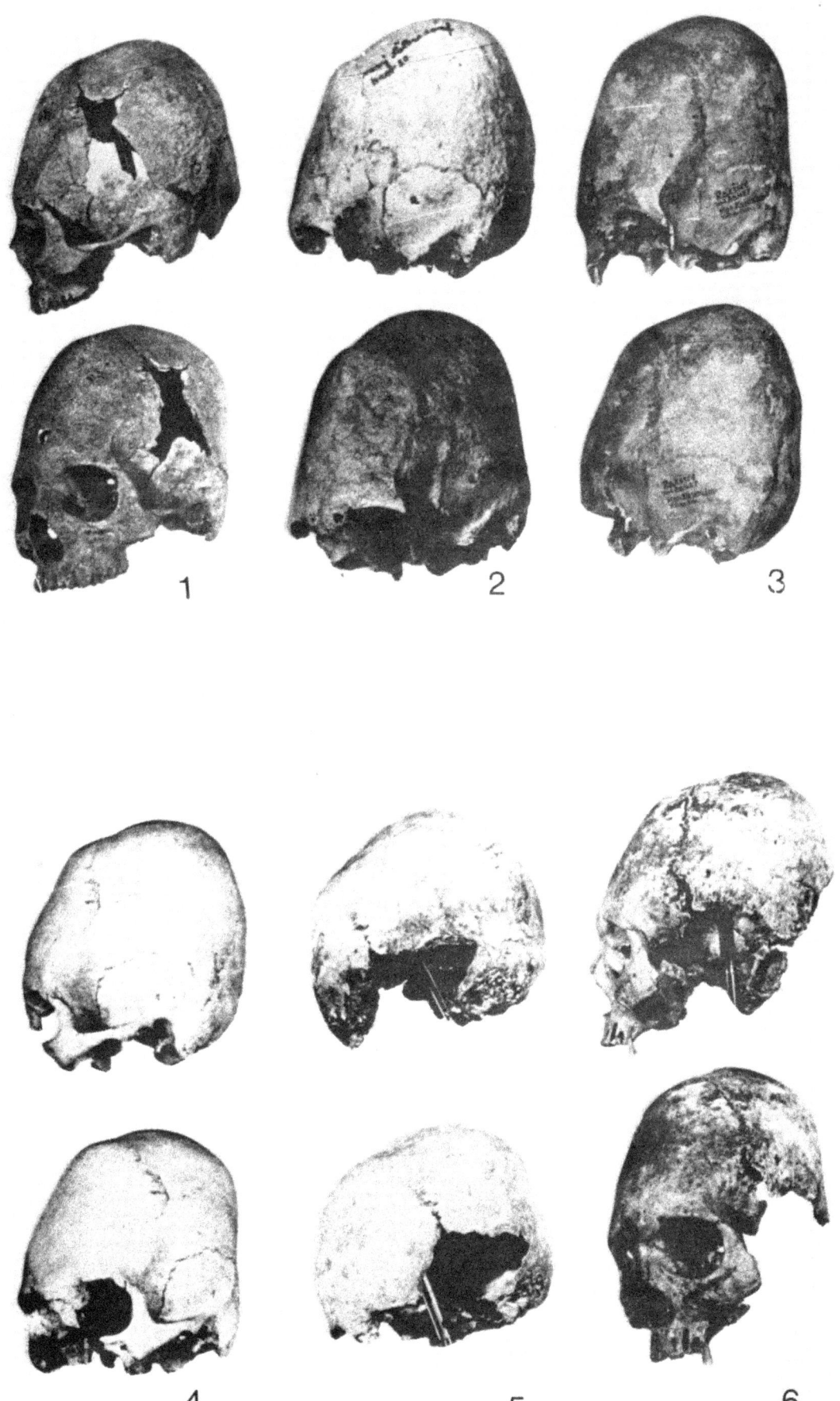

Fig. 27 Artificially formed skulls from Moravia.
1. Novy Saldorf, grave X_4; 2. Novy Saldorf, grave 30;
3. Raksice; 4. Nakló; 5. Slapanice; 6. Staré Mesto.

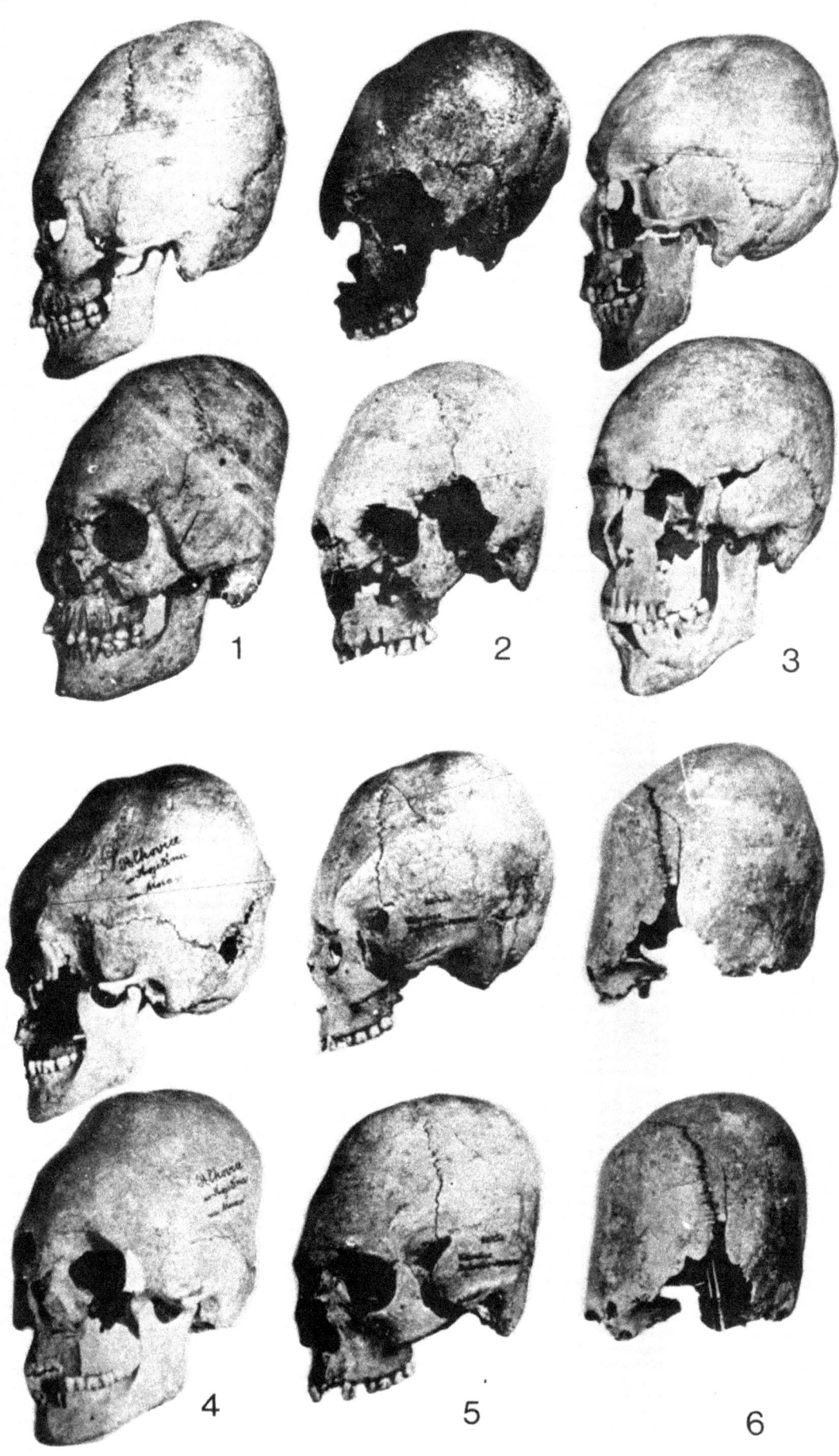

Fig. 28 Artificially formed skulls from Moravia.
1. Vacenovice; 2. Znojmo; 3. Sedlesovice; 4. Polkovice;
5. Vicemilice; 6. Nova Ves.

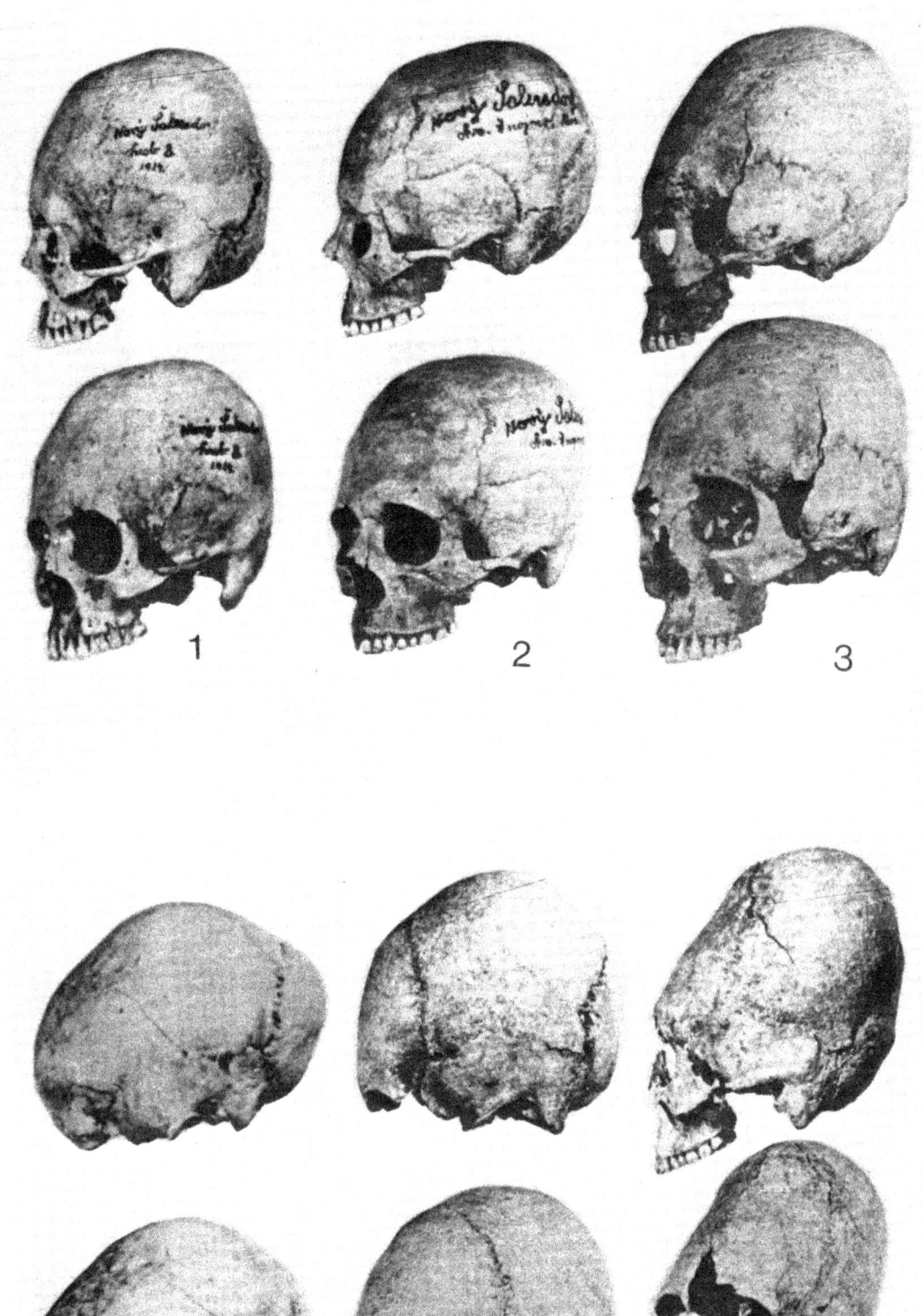

Fig. 29 Artificially formed skulls from Novy Saldorf, Moravia.
1. Grave 8; 2. Grave 8; 3. Grave X_2; 4. Grave X_6;
5. Grave X_5; 6. Grave X_3.

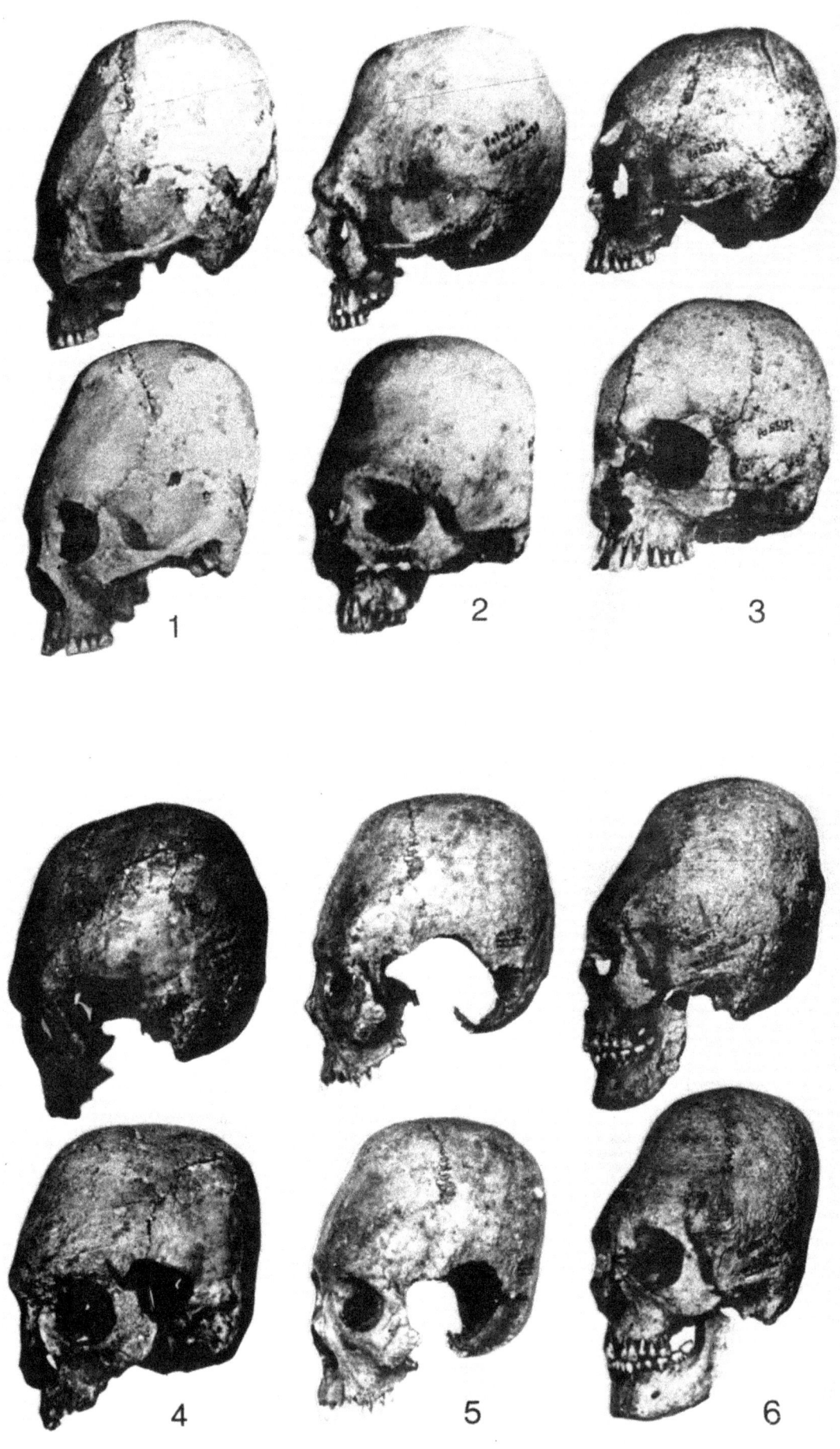

Fig. 30 Artificially formed skulls from Velatice, Moravia.
1. Grave X_4; 2. Grave X_1; 3. X_3; 4. X_1; 5. X_5; 6. X_6.

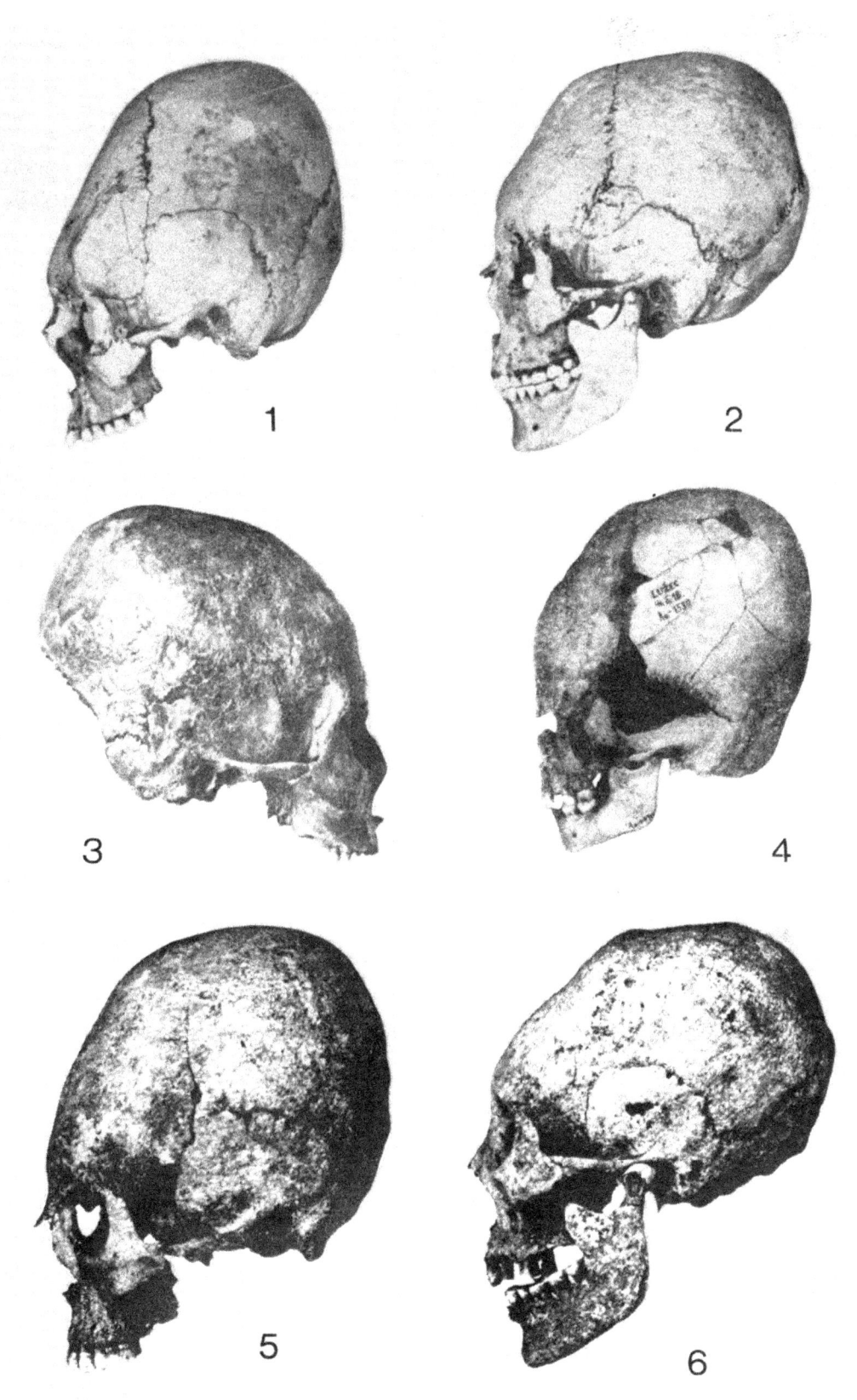

Fig. 31 Artificially formed skulls from Czechoslovakia.
1. Vyskov, grave 42; 2. Vyskov, grave 35; 3. Klucov, grave 1;
4. Luzec, grave 18; 5. Celakovice; 6. Celakovice.

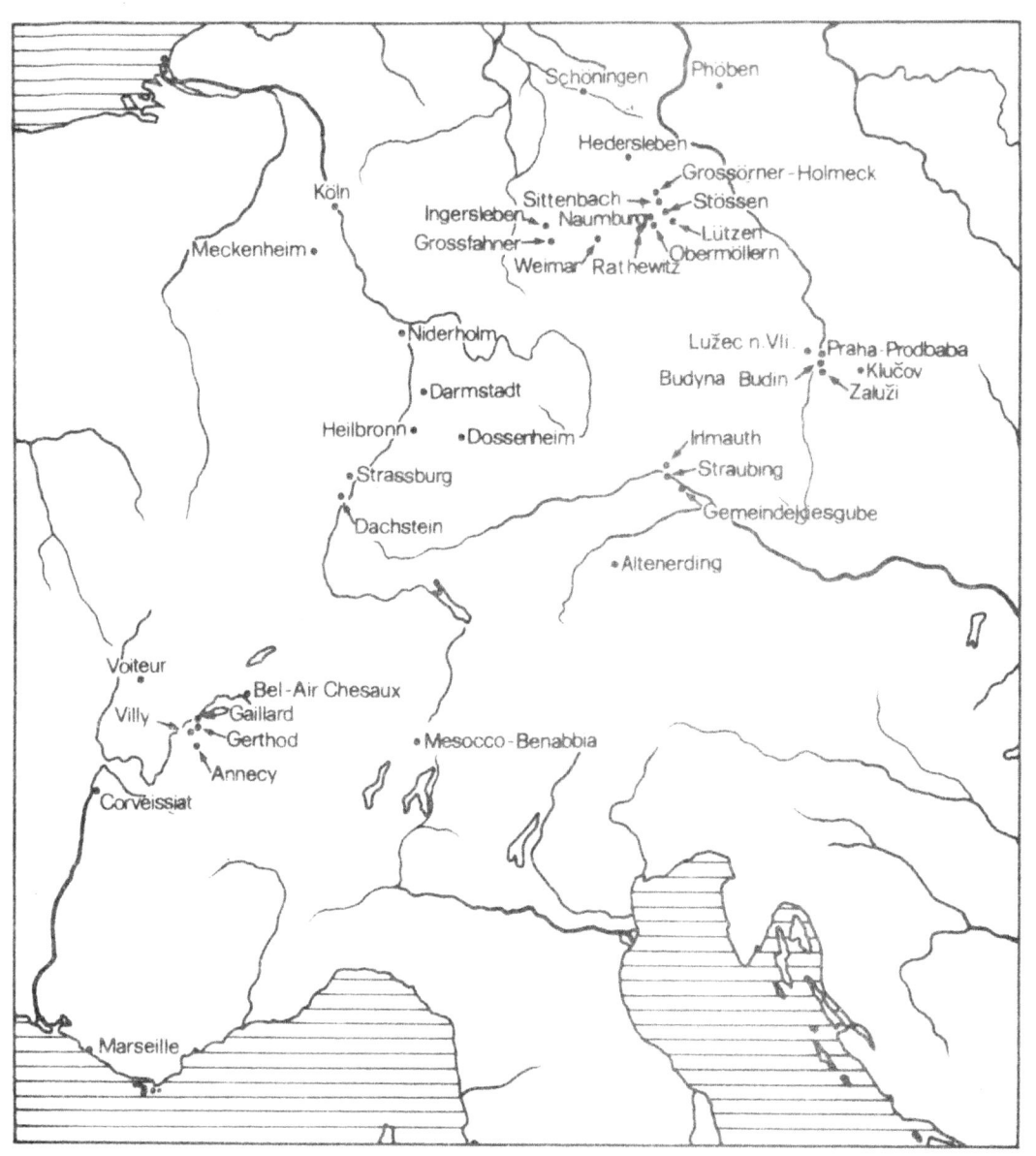

Fig. 32 Sites in Central and Western Europe where artificially formed skulls have been found.

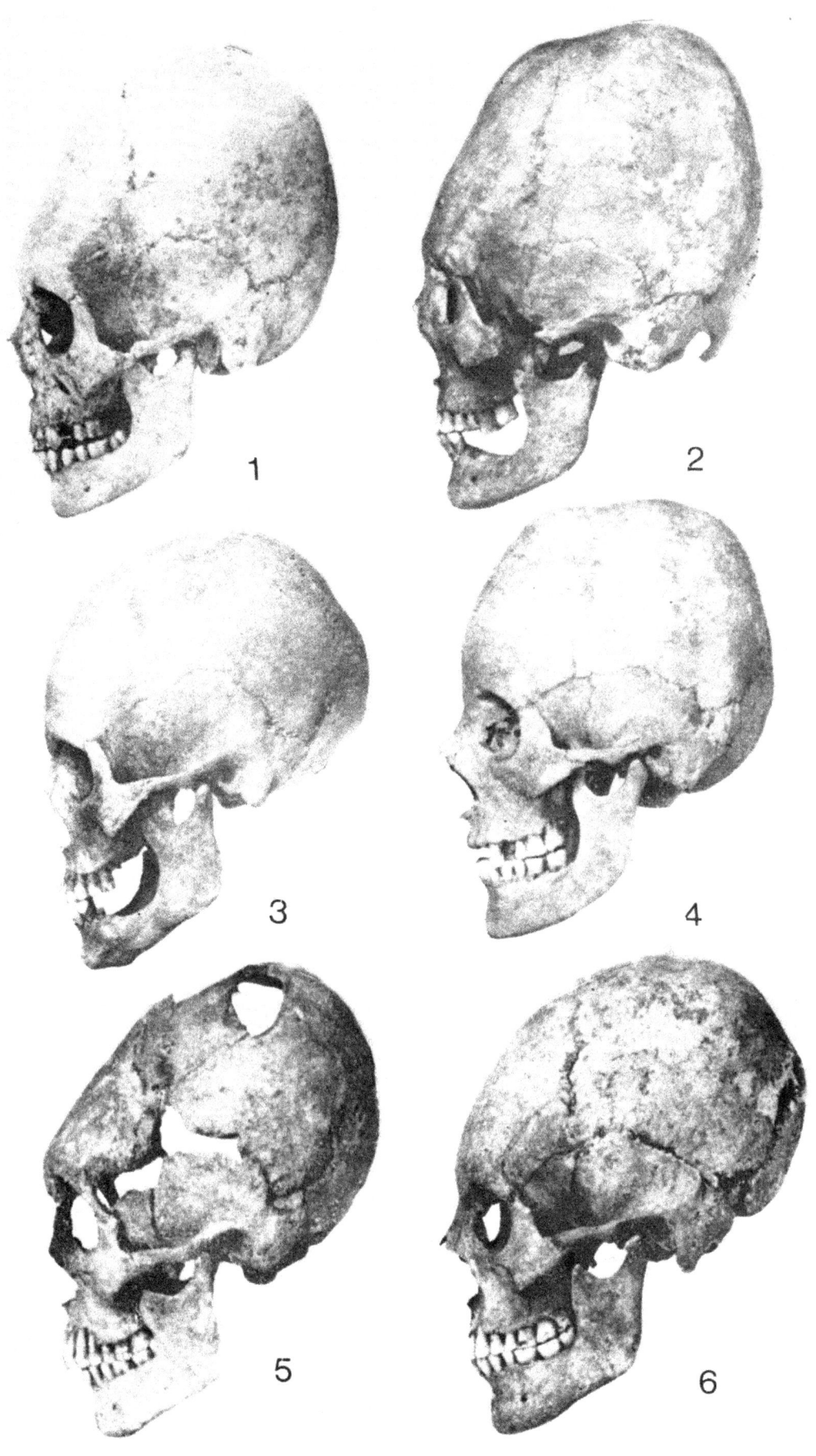

Fig. 33 Artificially formed skulls from Germany.
1. Hedersleben; 2. Obermöllern; 3. Sittichenbach, grave 20; 4. Rathewitz; 5. Lutzen; 6. Ingersleben.

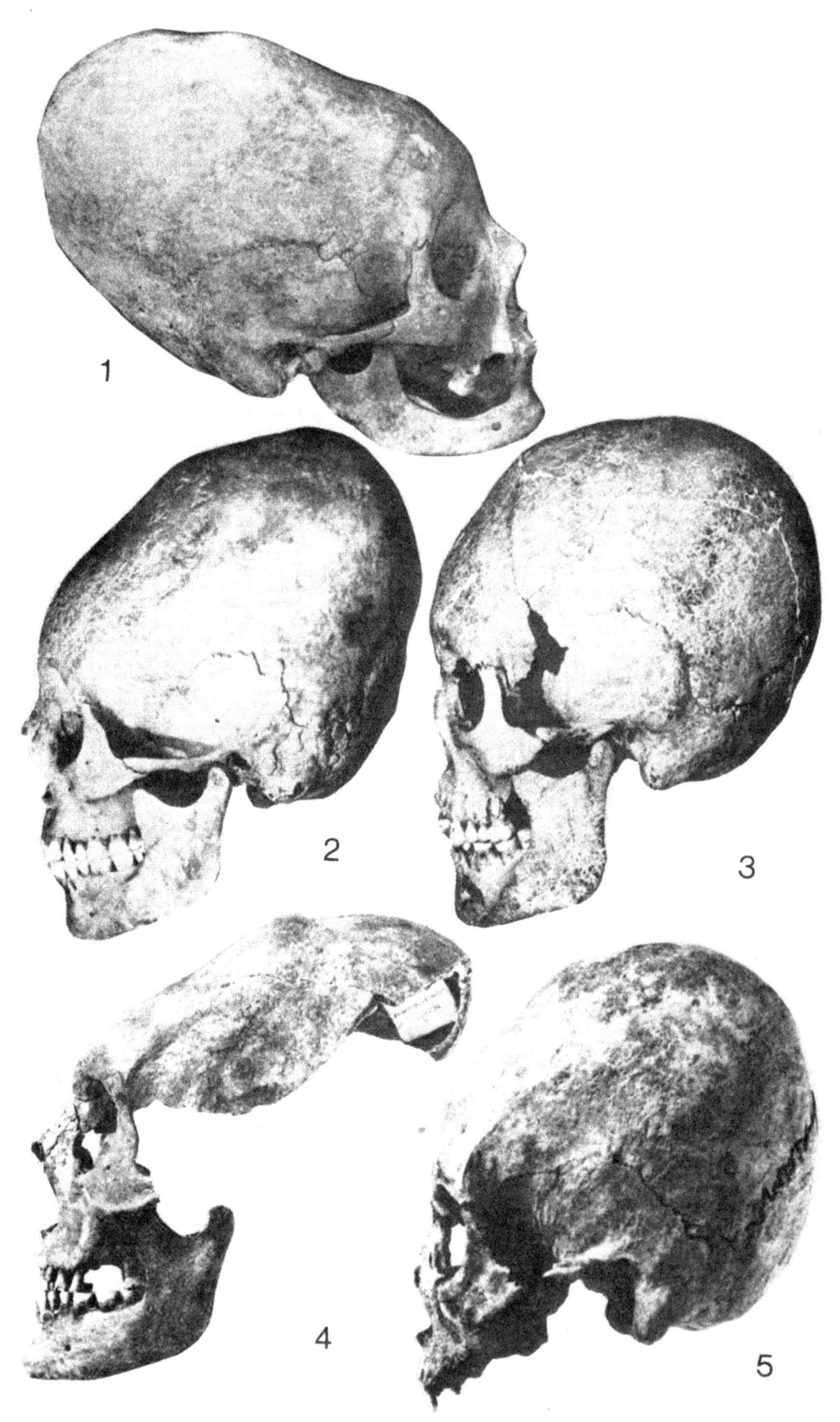

Fig. 34 Artificially formed skulls from Germany.
1. Dossenheim; 2. Altenerding; grave 513; 3. Altenerding, grave 125; 4. Eltheim, grave 172; 5. Irlmauth, grave 253.

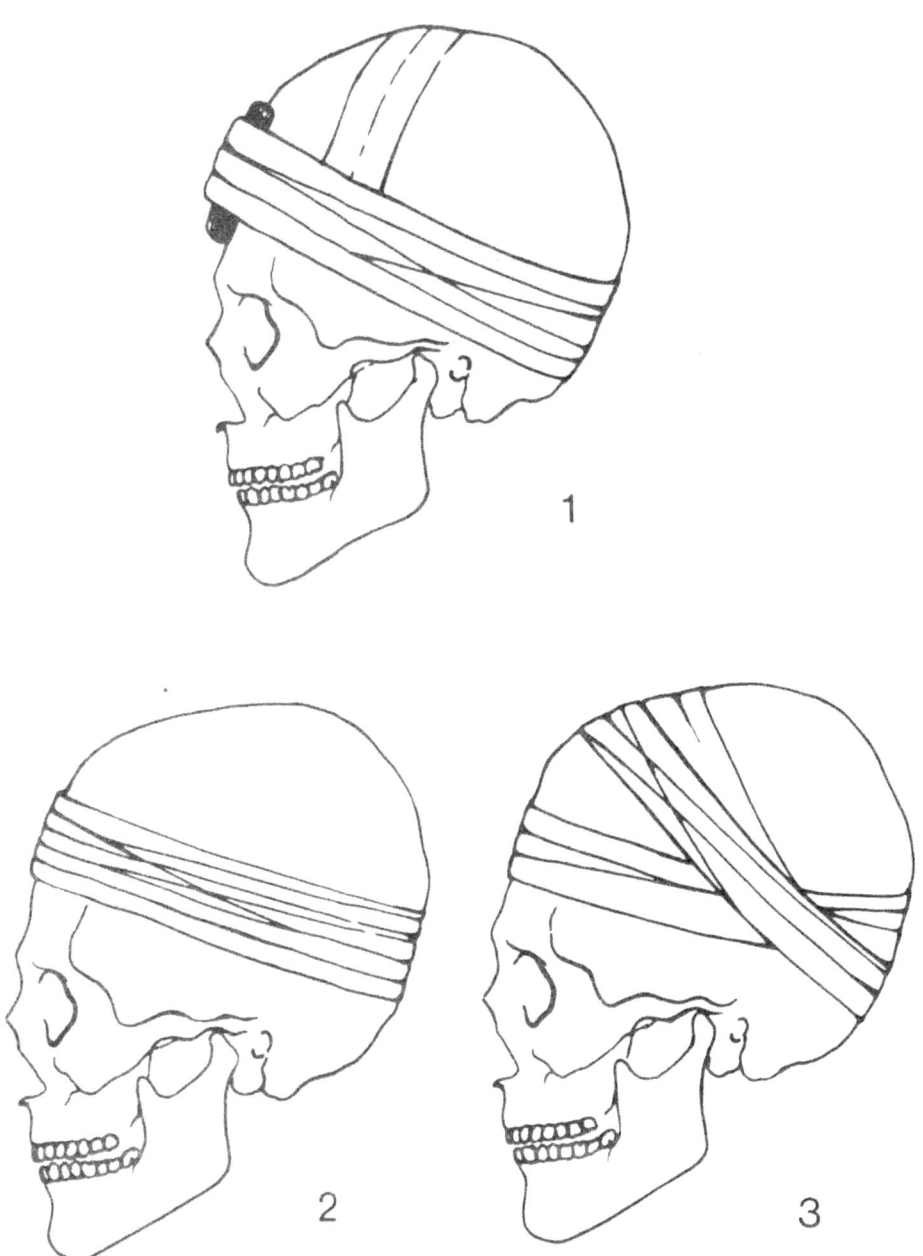

Fig. 35 Methods of artificially forming the skulls of newborn children used in Eurasia. 1. The "forehead-pillow"; 2. Simple bandaging; 3. Double bandaging.

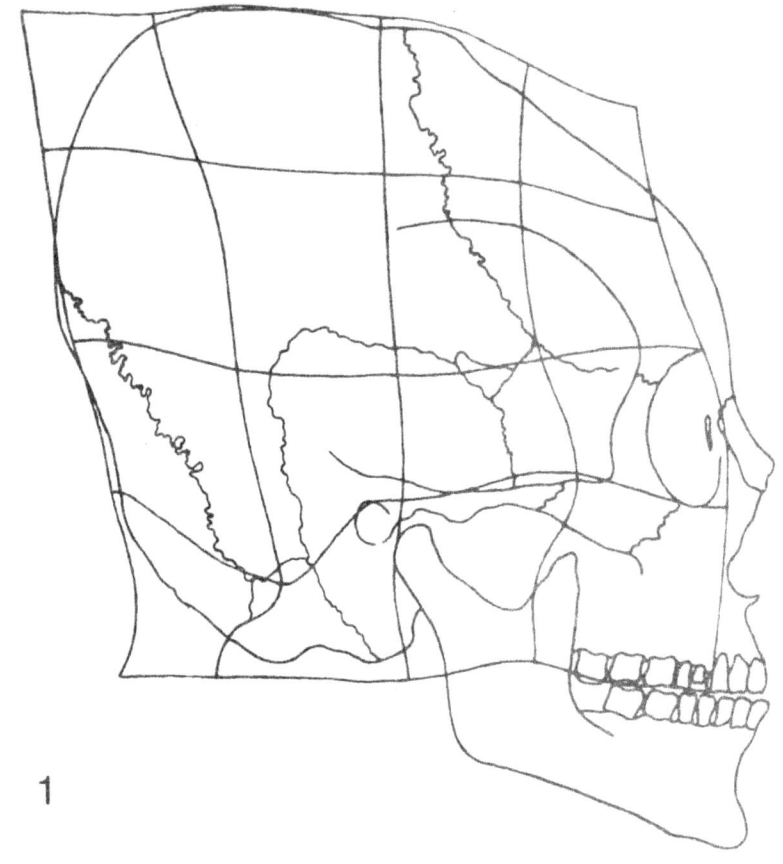

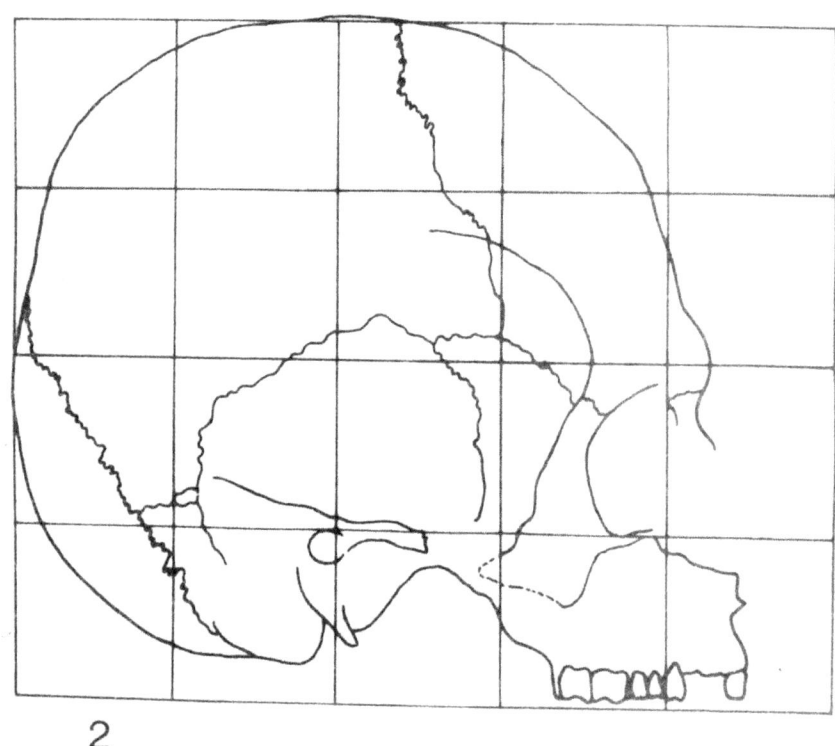

Fig. 36 Skull changes arising from artificial cranial formation (after H. Hellmuth).

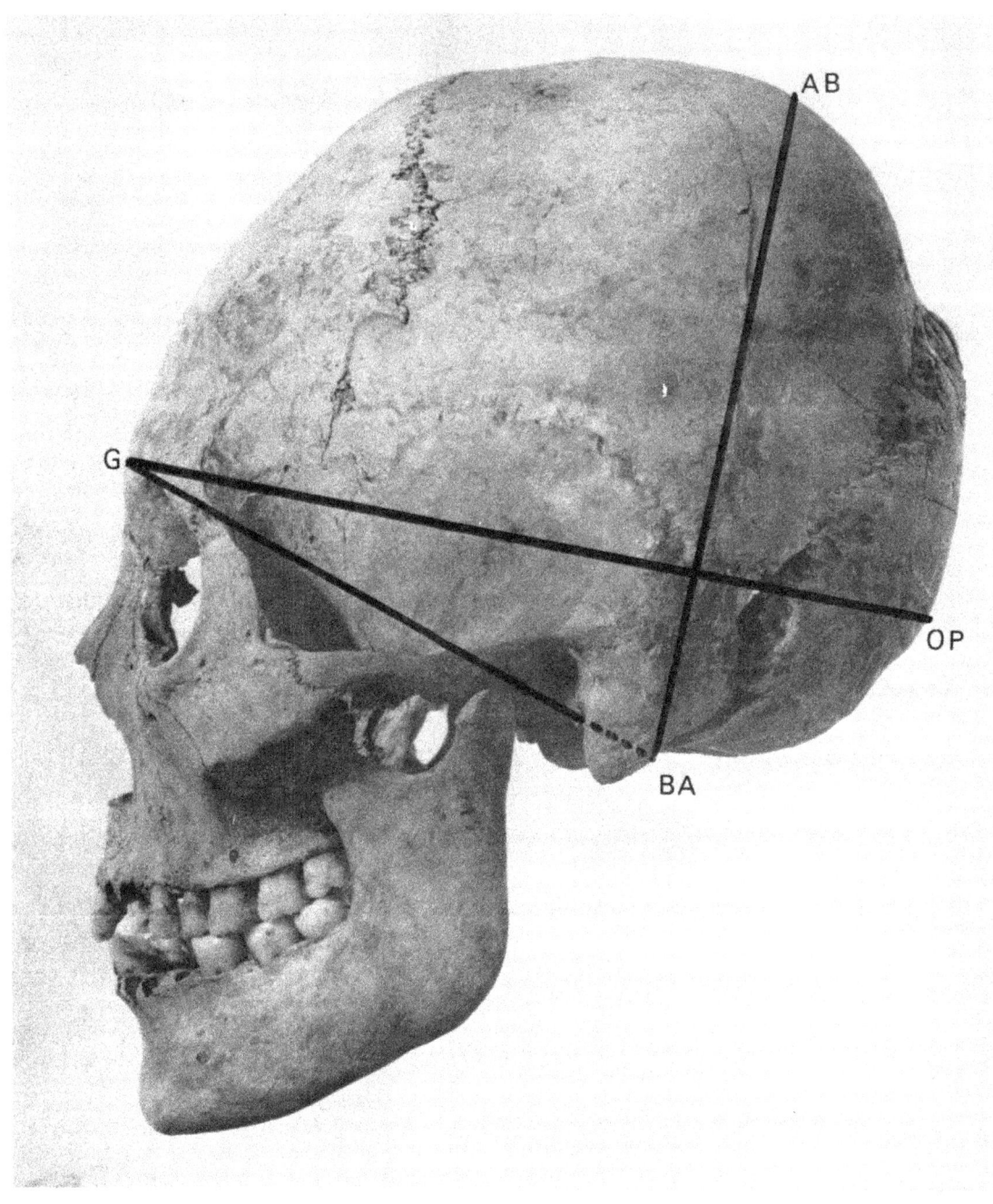

Fig. 37 Measurements taken to determine the extent of cranial formation.
BA = basion; AB = antibasion; G = glabella; OP = opisthion.

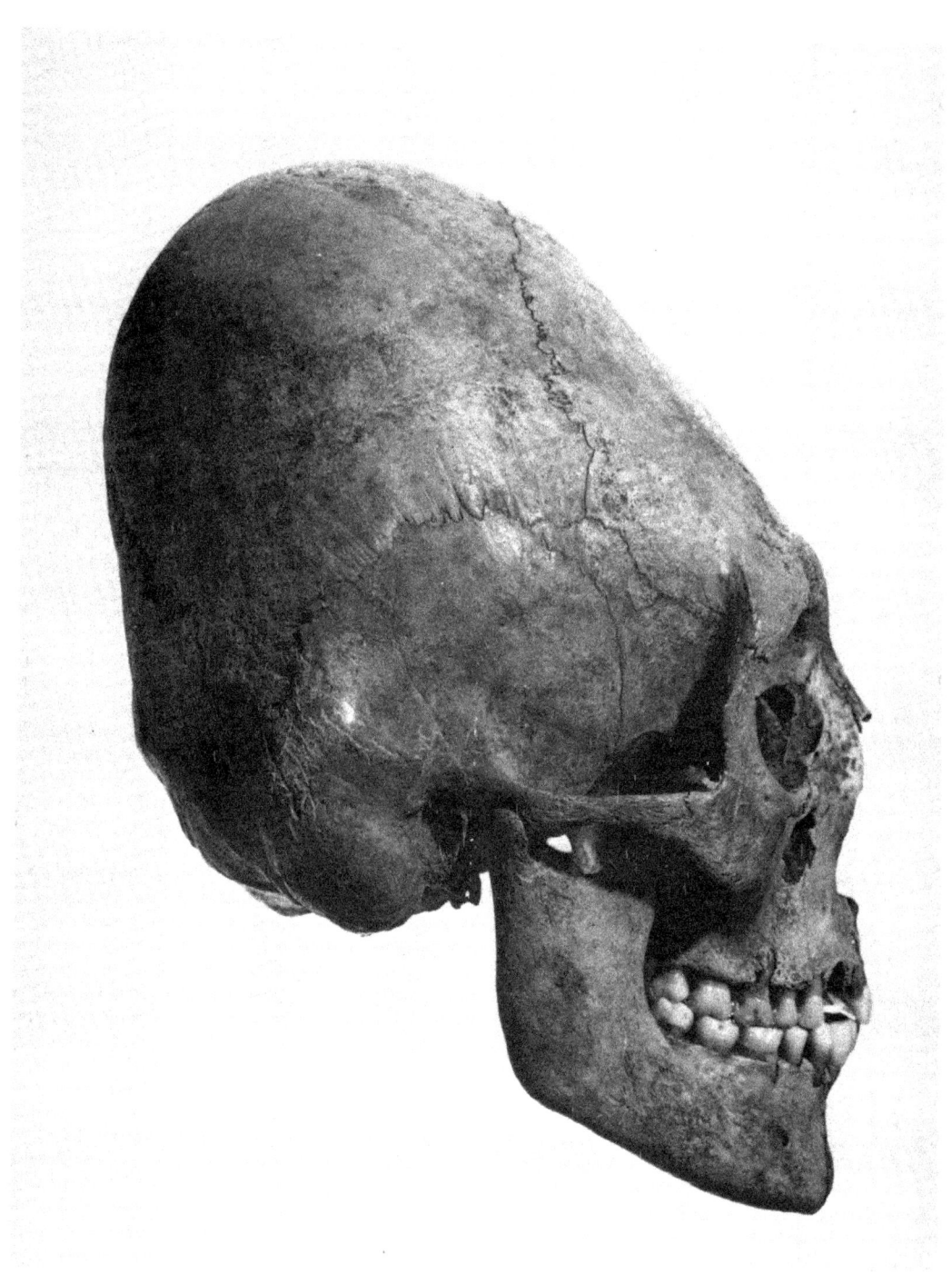

Fig. 38 Artificially formed skull from Hács-Béndekpuszta (Hungary), grave 23.

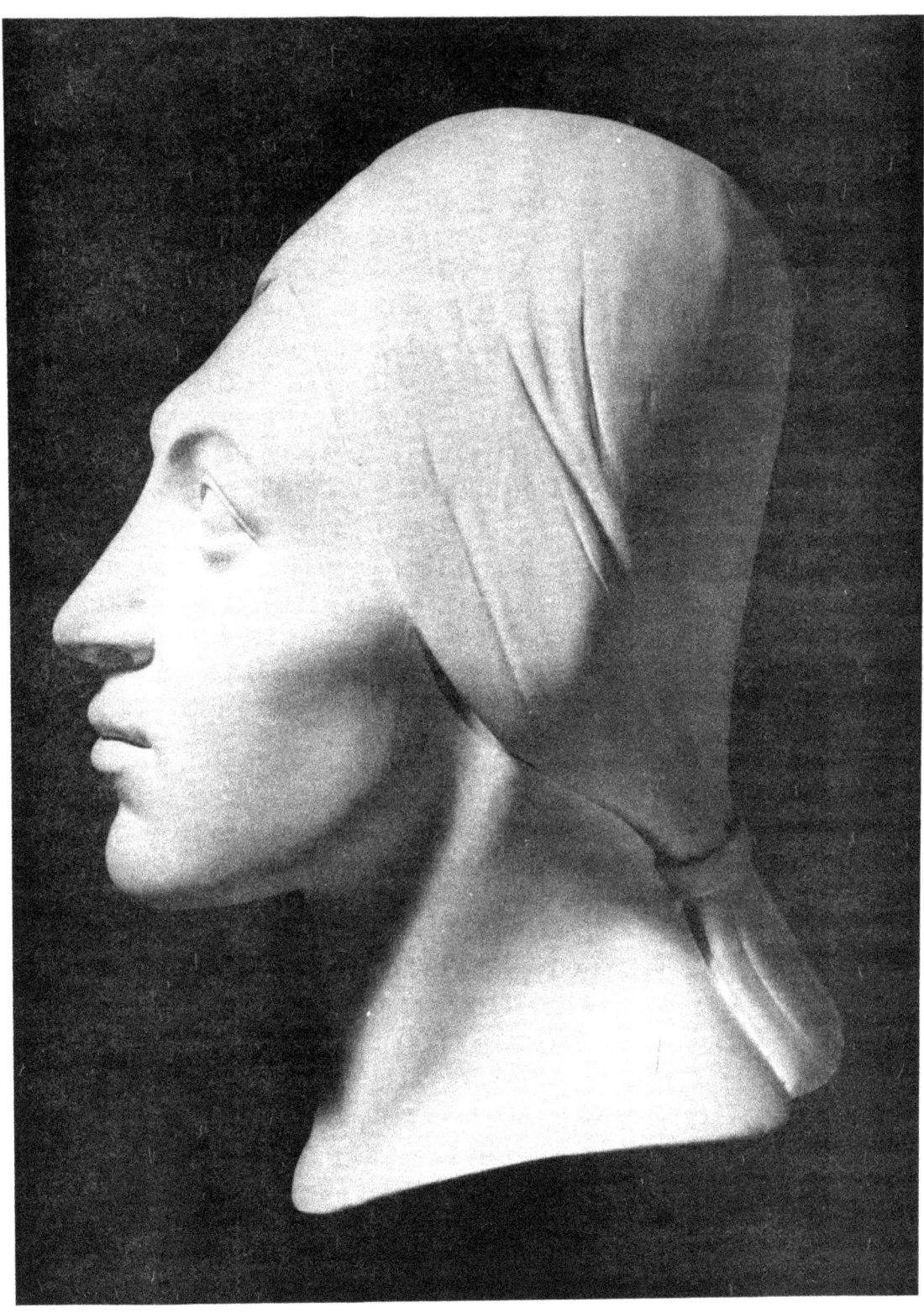

Fig. 39 The reconstruction of the face of the artificially formed skull from Hács-Béndekpuszta (Hungary), grave 23. Reconstruction by Károly Arpás.

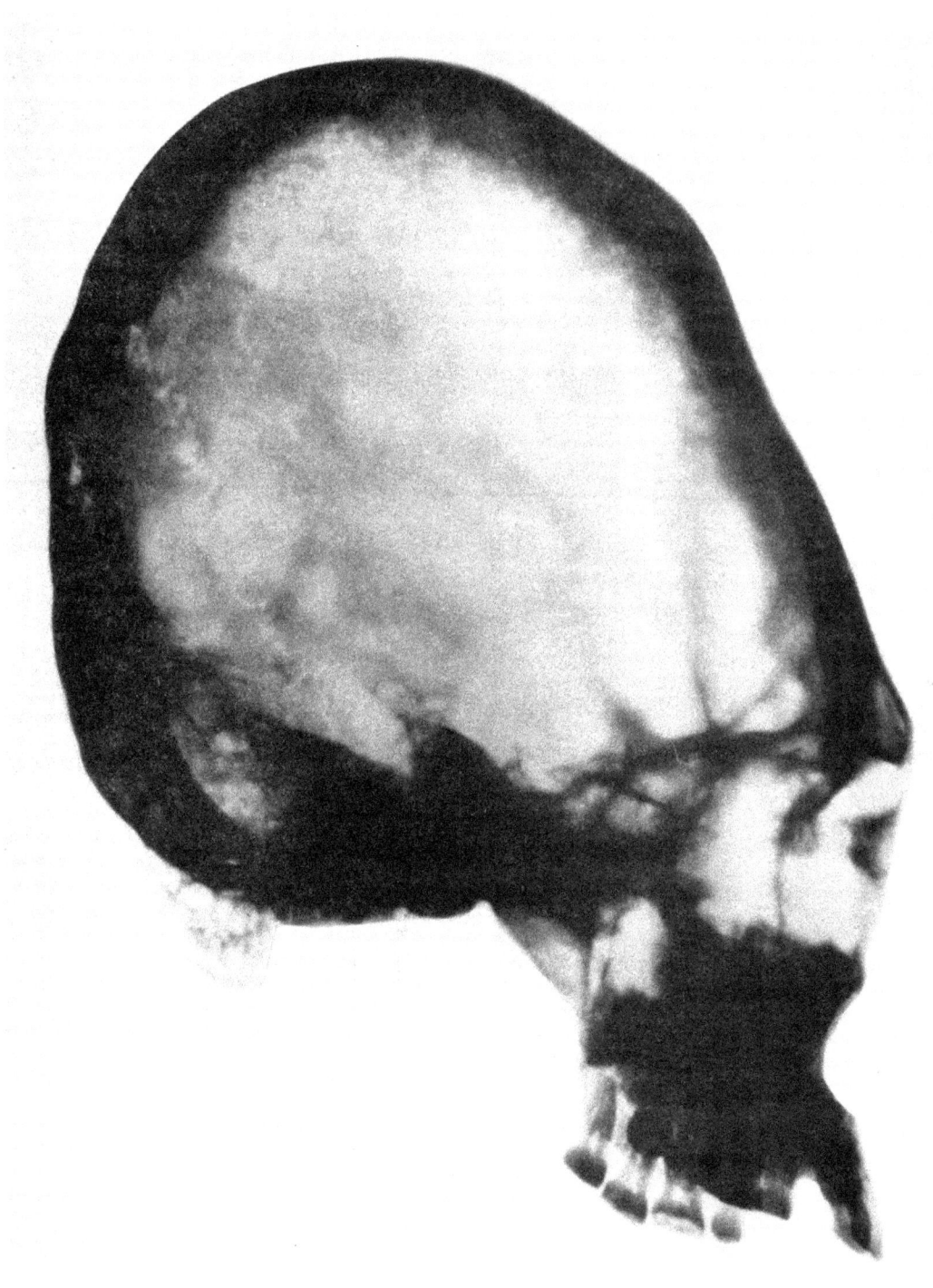

Fig. 40 X-ray photograph of the artificially formed skull from Tamási-Adorjánpuszta, Hungary. The areas where the bandages restricted the wall of the cranium can clearly be seen.

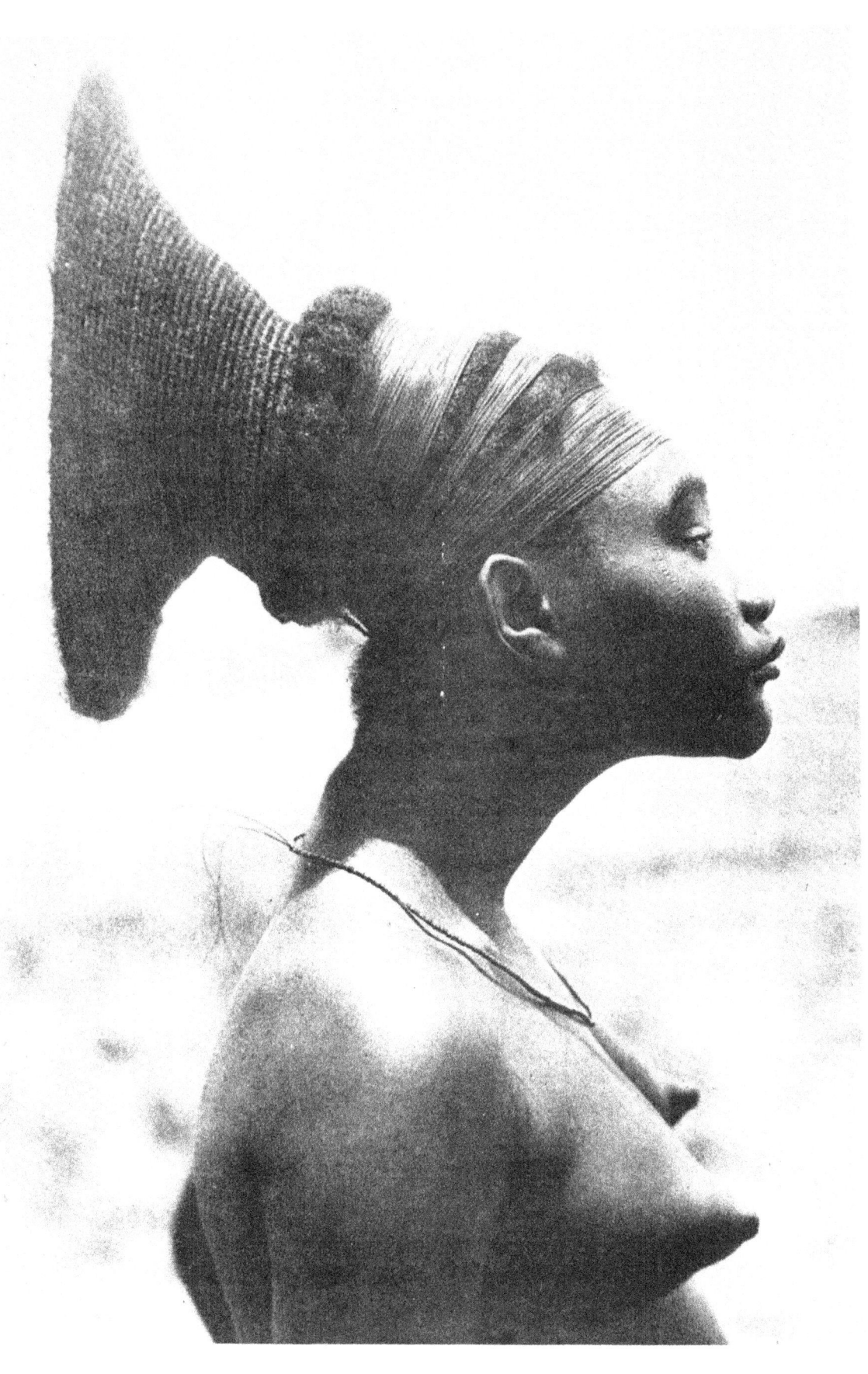

Fig. 41 A Mangbetu woman with artificially formed head (H. Bernatzik).

www.ingramcontent.com/pod-product-compliance
Ingram Content Group UK Ltd.
Pitfield, Milton Keynes, MK11 3LW, UK
UKHW060200240426
12048UKWH00029B/1665

9 780860 540298